Sérgio Valverde Marques dos Santos
Rita de Cássia de Marchi Barcellos Dalri
Fábio de Souza Terra

Self-Esteem, Stress and Accidents at Work in Nursing

Sérgio Valverde Marques dos Santos
Rita de Cássia de Marchi Barcellos Dalri
Fábio de Souza Terra

Self-Esteem, Stress and Accidents at Work in Nursing

An analysis of hospital environments

ScienciaScripts

Imprint

Any brand names and product names mentioned in this book are subject to trademark, brand or patent protection and are trademarks or registered trademarks of their respective holders. The use of brand names, product names, common names, trade names, product descriptions etc. even without a particular marking in this work is in no way to be construed to mean that such names may be regarded as unrestricted in respect of trademark and brand protection legislation and could thus be used by anyone.

Cover image: www.ingimage.com

This book is a translation from the original published under ISBN 978-613-9-69522-5.

Publisher:
Sciencia Scripts
is a trademark of
Dodo Books Indian Ocean Ltd. and OmniScriptum S.R.L publishing group

120 High Road, East Finchley, London, N2 9ED, United Kingdom
Str. Armeneasca 28/1, office 1, Chisinau MD-2012, Republic of Moldova, Europe
Printed at: see last page
ISBN: 978-620-7-01852-9

SUMMARY

Chapter 1	**6**
Chapter 2	**11**
Chapter 3	**17**
Chapter 4	**24**
Chapter 5	**29**
Chapter 6	**36**

INTRODUCTION

The contemporary world of work is undergoing profound transformations. Themes such as globalization, flexibility, competitiveness and new forms of work organization have a guaranteed place in the analyses of organizational scholars. In the phase known as the Third Industrial Revolution, the people who work in these places have become a source of greater interest, as they enable organizations to gain a competitive advantage. These transformations generate a complex environment, marked by technological and scientific advances, changes in concepts, values and paradigm shifts that guide all segments of society (PIRES; MACEDO, 2006).

The situation mentioned above can be better understood by analyzing the consequences of the transformations that have taken place in the world of work. Since the 1970s, the working class has suffered great damage to its organization and hard-won rights. This damage was caused by the process of restructuring production and the incorporation of neoliberal ideas by the states, both in the central and peripheral economies. In Brazil, these events occurred in a unique and belated way, starting in the 1980s (SOUZA E SILVA, 2008).

The transformations that took place in the world of work at the turn of the 20th to the 21st century were remarkable and the worldwide growth in unemployment is certainly the most perverse aspect of this situation. Despite all the scientific and technological development, all the important innovations in the technical basis of production processes, there has been little relief from human toil. In fact, these changes in the economy and society as a whole, resulting from productive restructuring, which became more visible in the 1990s, ended up intensifying the exploitation of the workforce and making employment more precarious (NAVARRO; PADILHA, 2007).

In the competitive world of work, where there is a greater demand for new technologies, industry is growing at an unprecedented rate. Unlike all past revolutions, these new technologies are increasingly agile and flexible and are changing not only industries, but also society, politics, the public sector and the economy. It is in this context that the fourth industrial revolution is taking place. This new concept encompasses the main technological innovations: automation, control and information technology, based on Cyber-Physical Systems, the Internet of Things and the Internet of Services (BRITO, 2017).

With the transformations that have taken place in the world of work in the 21st century, workers have become more demanding in the workplace, increasing their physical and psychological load. As a result, the number of accidents recorded in the workplace has grown. In 2010 there were 709,974 accidents at work in Brazil, while in 2013 this number rose to 717,911 (KAMIMURA, TAVARES, 2012; BRASIL, 2013).

Work can often be seen as a factor that causes changes in the living conditions, illness and death of human beings. Thus, work itself, which values and dignifies man, can cause suffering and illness when not carried out in suitable conditions, which do not favor the psychophysiological capacities of individuals, especially those who work in the health sector, such as nursing professionals (MARZIALE, 2010).

It is important to emphasize that health is not seen as a simplistic concept of the absence of disease, but is also determined by the varied external influences of the environment, as well as the lifestyle of individuals and the balance between external and internal human factors. It is believed that this balance is closely related to the harmony between all the vital areas that surround the worker, as seen in the concept of the World Health Organization (WHO) in 1948, and is directly associated with quality of life (THE WHOQOL GROUP, 1995).

In this context, the term quality of life has been inserted into the workplace, where workers spend a large part of their time. The competitiveness and demands of the job market, often promoted by technological and scientific advances, define the worker as a powerhouse. Commitment and motivation become the fuel for this power. Promoting quality of life in the workplace has therefore become essential to maintaining workers' motivation and commitment. This factor becomes even more important when it comes to hospital nursing professionals (ALVES, 2011).

With the aim of improving the well-being and safety of workers, reducing losses due to absenteeism, accidents at work and medical assistance, some Brazilian institutes have been adapting US program models aimed at improving the quality of life of workers, through a holistic vision (SILVA; LIMA, 2007).

With regard to the work process in hospital nursing services, it is worth noting that this process has characteristics that stem from the way it is organized and developed. However, the superimposition of specific workloads on workers has a significant impact on their physical and mental health. The activities carried out by nursing workers lead to exposure to occupational risks and wear and tear, which reflect on the health-disease process and can worsen over time, determining physical and psychosocial inadequacies, including changes in self-esteem, stress and the occurrence of accidents at work (SECCO et al., 2010).

It should be emphasized that nursing staff are exposed to a variety of occupational risks when carrying out their work activities. These risks can influence their working practices, contributing to the onset of illnesses, including psychiatric illnesses and/or accidents at work. These occurrences can interfere with workers' well-being, their daily lives and, consequently, their work activities (BORSOI; CODO, 1995; CAMPBELL; MUPHY; HURREL, 1997; CARAN, 2007).

Most nursing workers work in hospitals. These work environments expose them to occupational risks, double working hours, hostile and stressful environments and, consequently, accidents at work. In this respect, it is worth mentioning that when workers are involved in accidents or suffer from their work, they can develop a self-reproach in relation to their work activities. In this way, they are exposed to emotional suffering factors such as fear, anguish, negative self-assessment, embarrassment and judgment, which in turn can increase stress and reduce their level of self-esteem and quality of life (MICHEL, 2000; SECCO et al., 2010; SILVA, 2012; VARGAS; DANTAS; GOIS, 2005).

Ronsein et al., (2004), states that the importance of psychosomatic stressors is widely recognized, being as potent as microorganisms or unhealthy conditions in triggering illnesses.

Research by Prochaska et al. (2011) found that a significant proportion of workers' loss of productivity was related to emotional problems, reducing their performance by almost 36%. National and international studies have shown the occurrence of accidents at work among nursing professionals and their exposure to psychic damage, such as anxiety, depression, stress and low self-esteem (PROCHASKA et al., 2011; BEZERRA et al., 2015).

In the organizational context of the hospital environment, stressed nursing staff are more susceptible to accidents at work and occupational illnesses. In addition, they may carry out their activities inefficiently, disorganize their work, become dissatisfied and decrease productivity, which will certainly result in consequences for the individual and/or the population they assist (FARIAS; MAURO; ZEITONE, 2000).

Occupational stress is the result of the interaction between working conditions and the characteristics of the worker, in which the demands of the job exceed their abilities to cope with them. Excessive tension, culminating in long working hours, is among the main stress factors for Brazilian professionals, with 70% of the economically active population suffering sequelae due to high levels of tension. The lack of information and awareness of the level of stress has contributed to worsening the situation (ROSSI; MEURS; PERREWE, 2013).

It is therefore necessary to continually build up knowledge for hospital workers, including nurses. It is believed that this construction could bring about changes in the working environment, through the implementation of programs to prevent accidents at work and psychiatric illness, awareness of the use of individual and collective protective equipment and improved adherence to training on safe working practices. In this way, it will be possible to promote better care for users, as well as an appropriate quality of life and physical and mental health for nursing workers.

CHAPTER 1

Background to the nursing profession

The need to care for the sick has been with human beings since the dawn of time. In the beginning, temples, convents and monasteries received the sick and provided special care, with the aim of looking after the body as well as the soul of the sick person. This situation was particularly present in the Middle Ages, where the idea was shared that in cases of illness and other ailments, spiritual assistance was the most appropriate remedy (BELLATO; PASTI; TAKEDA, 1997).

In the 18th century, the hospital was considered to be an institution for caring for the poor, but it also served to separate and exclude them; the sick poor were considered dangerous because they often carried contagious diseases. For this reason, hospitals were built outside urban areas, mainly because of their social character. Activities in the hospitals were carried out by religious or lay people, usually women, who did the work with a view to saving their souls through charitable support (FOUCAULT, 1993).

Gradually, the hospital detached itself from religious influences, characterizing itself as a social institution for which the state was responsible. In this way, it was believed that hospitals could carry out effective therapeutic activities for inpatients if they overcame the unsanitary conditions of dirt and promiscuity, such as the use of collective beds where patients stayed together (ANTUNES, 1985).

According to Almeida (1984), at the end of the 18th century doctors began to occupy space in hospitals. However, the problems arising from the insalubrity within these institutions persisted until the middle of the 19th century, with the establishment of bacteriology by Pasteur and the concepts of asepsis by Lister. At the same time, the most important figure in the history of modern nursing emerged, Florence Nightingale, who brought new perspectives to the profession and to health care.

It is worth mentioning that nursing is an activity as old as mankind and was born out of the need to care for the sick. The history of nursing is present before, during and after the Middle Ages. In Greek society, before this period, nursing was practiced by slaves, priests and women in Greek society. For the primitives, the understanding of health and illness was linked to supernatural factors and the action of spirits. The Greeks, on the other hand, related health and illness to changes in mood and objective causes, and not only to supernatural factors (SILVA, 1989).

In the Christian and medieval periods, caring for the sick was seen as a kind and charitable activity. But this was done with the aim of saving the soul of both the sick person and the caregiver. This led to the emergence of deaconesses, whose ordination was aimed at providing a service that consisted of meeting the survival needs of sick and needy people (ANGERAMI; CORREIA, 1989).

However, care practices needed theoretical knowledge to underpin the activities. Thus, based on the Rules of St. Benedict, establishments were created to train people to work in care, with women's institutions standing out, which brought together religious women from the community who provided care for the sick (MELEK; ROCHA, 2008). Among these noblewomen was Saint Radegunda, who gave up the throne of France to found a convent for the treatment of lepers in the 16th century. Of the institutions created, the most notable in Germany was the Institute of Deaconesses of Kaiseaswith, and in France the Confraternity of the Daughters of Charity of St. Vincent de Paul (PAIXAO, 1979).

At the end of the 18th century, the religious model of nursing, which emerged in the Christian world and continued through the Middle Ages, came up against English capitalism. With the rise of the bourgeoisie as the dominant social class, nursing became an art or vocation. In this way, the religious model of nursing was replaced by the vocational one in capitalism (ALMEIDA; ROCHA, 1989).

In the Modern Age, nursing took two directions, one linked to Christian charity and vocation and the other to professionalization. However, these ideas remained empirical until the first half of the 19th century. With Florence Nightingale, in the second half of the 19th century, the nursing profession underwent radical transformations, through work based on scientific foundations, which supported its professional formation (BELLATO; PASTI; TAKEDA, 1997).

In 1854, Florence was invited by the British government to work in the military hospitals during the Crimean War. She managed to do an excellent job, reducing the number of deaths among the soldiers. In 1860, Florence created the Nightingale School at St. Thoma's Hospital, with the aim of preparing nurses to work in the nursing service (GIOVANINI, 1995).

Florence Nightingale constituted modern nursing, regulating hierarchy and discipline for nursing work, reflecting her high social class and her religious and military training. In this way, she materialized the relations of domination and subordinacy, reproducing the relations of social classes in nursing practice (ALMEIDA; ROCHA, 1989).

The entry of nursing into the hospital was due to the participation of Florence, who found precarious conditions for promoting the healing of patients in the hospital environment, due to the lack of hygiene and great promiscuity. In this way, she tried to standardize and regulate the organization of the patient's therapeutic environment. With this, he legitimized an institutional hierarchy, where he prepared nurses to head wards and superintendents. Thus, she instituted technical divisions of labor, whereby the *ladies nurses* who had high social positions were in charge of nursing administration, and the *nurses* who had lower social levels were responsible for nursing care (BELLATO; PASTI; TAKEDA, 1997).

In Brazil, nursing began in the colonial period. When the Jesuits introduced their customs into the lives of the Indians, they contributed to a disturbance in the physiological balance of the Indians' bodies, generating endemic and epidemic diseases (GIOVANINI, 1995). Thus, the Indians themselves took care of the sick in their tribe out of necessity. With colonization, this care also became the responsibility of Jesuits, religious, lay people, volunteers and slaves (TONINI; FLEMING, 2002).

In the middle of 1543, the first Santas Casas de Misericordia were founded. At this time, slaves and volunteers cared for the sick and were supervised by the religious, who also provided some assistance to the sick. This type of empirical nursing lasted from colonization until the beginning of the 20th century (TURKIEWICZ, 1995).

In the 19th century, nursing emerged in Brazil with Ana Justina Ferreira Neri, due to her outstanding work caring for soldiers during the Paraguayan War. For her tireless work assisting soldiers, she was decorated by the Brazilian government at the end of the war (TONINI; FLEMING, 2002).

It is worth noting that modern nursing was established in Brazil in 1923, with the creation of the Anna Nery Nursing School in Rio de Janeiro, which was based on the *Nightingalean* model and aimed to train professionals for Public Health, as health education agents. Later, in 1943, the Sao Paulo School of Nursing was created in Sao Paulo, attached to the Faculty of Medicine of the University of Sao Paulo (USP)

(OGUISSO; FREITAS, 2005).

From this time onwards, several graduate nurses began to gain prominence in Brazil and were considered pioneers of the nursing profession in the country. Taking care to build a history for the nursing profession with more scientific consistency allows professionals in the field to grow intensely and correctly, as well as being able to become more decisive and active (VITORIA REGIS; PORTO, 2006).

With the changes that took place in the middle of the 19th century, the hospital began to be seen as a place of healing. Doctors began to carry out their work in an attempt to cure the sick, sharing their space with nursing (TREVIZAN, 1988).

With the increasing complexity of the hospital and the introduction of nursing in this institution, the hospital became a service-providing company. As a result, the division of labor was greatly influenced by the main administrative models (BELLATO; PASTI; TAKEDA, 1997). In this way, the division of nursing work was organized into administrative and educational tasks, which were the responsibility of the nurses, and care tasks, which were the responsibility of the nursing assistants and technicians (FERRAZ, 1990).

According to the Secretariat of Labor Management and Health Education, the nursing team is highly represented in the labor market in Brazil, including nurses, technicians and nursing assistants. A survey of health workers carried out in 2008 showed that of the 2,846,788 workers, 1,243,804 were nursing staff, which represented 43.37% of all these workers (BRASIL, 2010). According to the Federal Nursing Council (COFEN), in 2011 the number of nursing workers registered with the Nursing Councils was 1,535,568 professionals. This highlights the representativeness of this class of workers in the country's health context (BRASIL, 2013).

Nursing work, in order to meet the needs of the population, is mainly characterized by being continuous, i.e. carried out around the clock, organized in fixed schedules with unusual or rotating hours, in a shift system, including night shifts. It usually involves extensive weekly working hours, including weekends and public holidays (BARBOZA et al., 2008).

The legislation recognizes as a nurse, the holder of this diploma awarded by an educational institution, under the terms of the Law; the holder of the diploma or certificate of obstetrician or obstetric nurse, awarded under the terms of the law; the holder of a nurse's diploma or certificate and the holder of an obstetric nurse's or midwife's diploma or certificate, or equivalent, awarded by a foreign school in accordance with the laws of the country, registered under a cultural exchange agreement or re-evaluated in Brazil as a nurse's, obstetric nurse's or midwife's diploma; those who, not covered by the preceding paragraphs, have obtained a nurse's diploma in accordance with the provisions of point "d" of art. 3. of Decree No. 50.387 of March 28, 1961 (BRASIL, 2007). This professional has the role of holder of knowledge and controller of the nursing work process, and it is up to the other workers in this profession to carry out delegated tasks (LEOPARDI, 1999).

Among the functions of health professionals, the continuous relationships with others stand out, which can influence the lifestyle of the caregiver, as well as being evaluated as stressful. The characteristics of nursing, as a profession, are associated with highly standardized, fragmented work, due to the division of tasks and techniques, with a shift system (rotation), as well as excessive responsibility and the need to expand technical and technological knowledge (GUIDO, 2003).

In view of the above, it should be noted that the nursing team has a great deal of responsibility in hospital institutions for providing continuous care to patients. It is therefore necessary to provide comprehensive care for these professionals, by promoting workers' health, preventing accidents at work, psychiatric illness and better control of the occupational risks present in this work activity.

CHAPTER 2

Workers' health and occupational risks in nursing

The practice of work carried out by man refers to the transformation of nature and of himself, with the aim of obtaining a useful object, with work being the main element, the object to be transformed and the tools needed for this transformation (LAURELL; NORIEGA, 1989). As well as being indispensable for the maintenance of human life, work is fundamental for defining the health conditions of each person, since the moment of work becomes a privileged moment for the realization of the human being as a being aware of their own essence and their temporality (MERLO, 1991).

For Marziale (2010), work is seen as a factor that causes changes in the living conditions, illness and death of human beings. Thus, the very work that values and dignifies man can cause suffering and illness when not carried out under suitable conditions.

In an expanded concept described by the Ministry of Health, it is possible to state that Workers' Health is a field of knowledge that seeks to encompass the relationship between the health-disease process and work. Health and illness are considered to be a dynamic process linked to the models of productive development of the human being at historical moments (BRASIL, 2002).

In addition, the term Workers' Health is defined as a set of activities aimed at promoting the health of workers through health and epidemiological surveillance support. In this way, it aims to recover and rehabilitate the health of professionals subjected to the risks and/or problems caused by working conditions (BRASIL, 2006).

The purpose of Workers' Health is focused on the multidisciplinary and intersectoral approach of acting from the perspective of totality. In this way, it aims to overcome fragmented and watertight understanding and interventions, enabling workers to participate in the construction of knowledge about the impact of work on the health-disease process. In this way, they are able to interfere politically and promote health at work, while being considered subjects of their own lives and health (MARZIALE, 2010).

At the beginning of the 1970s, Brazilian hospitals began to worry about the health of their workers. A study showed that in 1971 there were 4,468 accidents at work in hospitals in Brazil. This led to the need to implement preventive methods to control accidents and occupational risks (GOMES, 1974). According to data from the Ministry of Social Security on the occurrence of accidents at work among health professionals, 51,417 accidents were recorded in hospital environments in 2011 (BRASIL, 2012).

It's worth pointing out that strategies aimed at workers' health need to be made clear to all professionals, especially nurses. Since these professionals work in the areas of public and hospital health, they can help to prevent accidents at work and their consequences for health. This support can help to reduce the statistics related to accidents at work, which are constantly present in the lives of the Brazilian population (SILVA, 2012).

According to the *National Institute for Occupational Safety and Health* (NIOSH) (1988), hospital environments have been considered unhealthy since ancient times because they offer procedures that put workers at risk of accidents, contact with occupational hazards and the occurrence of diseases. In addition, they are home to various infectious and contagious diseases brought in by patients, putting the health of professionals at risk. It is therefore believed that workers exposed to these risks need information and training to avoid and prevent health problems and accidents at work.

According to Baptista (2004), the health problems and illnesses caused by work should not only be understood as biophysical elements. Furthermore, the way people get sick and die should not only be seen as a natural phenomenon, but also as a socially determined event. In addition, in order to understand the determinants of illnesses and diseases that affect workers' health, ideological, political and cultural aspects must be analyzed, and not just the technical point of view of how work is carried out. This is because, according to the cultural and ideological formation of the worker, it will be determined how they react to the aggressions they suffer at work.

In the hospital environment, nurses work in the care process, providing direct and comprehensive care to patients. As a result, workers make continuous use of sharp and piercing objects, as well as handling biological materials. These factors contribute to the professional being exposed to occupational risks, such as physical, chemical, ergonomic, psychosocial and biological risks, which can be considered the main factors responsible for exposing health professionals to unhealthy situations

(BORSOI; CODO, 1995).

Analyzing occupational risks helps to identify potential sources of harm that can compromise workers' health and to promote preventive safety measures. Risk is therefore a basic component of prevention measures in health, epidemiology and Workers' Health (NUNES, 2009).

In this area of occupational risks, it is worth noting that they are characterized according to their specific characteristics. Physical risks are characterized by the forms of energy that expose workers to them, such as noise, abnormal pressure, vibration, radiation, extreme temperatures and lighting. Chemical risks are known as exposure to solid, liquid or gaseous substances, composed of chemical products capable of penetrating the body. Ergonomic risks are those related to man's adaptation to work, especially aspects related to inappropriate postures, materials, furniture, equipment and work organization, where the worker's psychophysiological characteristics are not taken into account (BRASIL, 1994; MARZIALE, 1995).

Psychosocial risk is understood as any psychic risk factor or agent present in the workplace. This risk can cause damage to the worker's mental/psychic health and is associated with the stresses of daily life, including those arising from work (CARAN, 2007). According to Barreto (2003), for the European Agency for Safety and Health at Work, psychosocial risks are subjective perceptions created by the professional in the organization of work. This issue can be identified through statistical data related to subjective judgments that affect the psychic area, morals, intellect, among others.

According to Campbell, Muphy and Hurrel (1997), workers are exposed to psychosocial risks depending on the type of work they do, such as jobs with little control over the worker or work methods; jobs with no decision-making role; monotonous and repetitive tasks; machine operation; excessive demands; payment linked to the performance of tasks; work that does not make use of the worker's potential; among others.

Often, the lack of recognition for nursing professionals is compounded by the high demands to which these workers are subjected. This factor may be related to both the competitiveness of the job market and the demands of the positions held. In this way, it is clear that these conditions can contribute to the manifestation of psychic illnesses in workers (VIEIRA et al., 2013).

In this context, some factors may be associated with psychosocial risks in the workplace, such as lack of training and preparation, long working hours, excessive workloads, fast work rhythms, subordinate work, conflict between teams, pressure from managers and colleagues, tension, stressful situations, lack of communication, dissatisfaction, fatigue, difficulty reconciling family and work, lack of autonomy and creativity, among others (CAMELO; ANGERAMI, 2007; LAURELL; NORIEGA, 1989; SILVA, 1996).

Still related to the idea of psychosocial risk, Caran (2007) states that there are emotional stressors, which are linked to competitiveness, insecurity, lack of recognition, fear of ridicule, lack of autonomy, absence of dialogue and respect and conflicts. Interpersonal relationships, with the imposition of inadequate leadership, confusing and contradictory activities, and organizational culture also stand out. Finally, it is necessary to add work-related stressors, such as excessive workload, scarcity of work, intensification of the pace of work and new demands, repetitiveness and emptying of the content of the task, bureaucratic work.

A problem faced by many nursing professionals in institutions is work overload. This is an important factor, since it can affect interpersonal relationships between workers in a way that encourages demotivation and can also contribute to dehumanized nursing care (OLIVEIRA et al., 2013).

It is important to emphasize that psychosocial risks are capable of damaging both the worker and the entire society in which he or she is inserted. These risks, among the various occupational risks at work, are attributed to factors such as the intensity of the mental load, the high degree of responsibility and the complexity of the task. In this way, they can lead to changes in the individual's mental health, caused by the stresses of daily life and other factors. These risks can lead to changes in the worker's health, such as anxiety, neurosis, sleep disorders, depression, stress and *Burnout* Syndrome, family conflicts, changes in self-esteem, violent attitudes, among others (CARAN, 2007; FACTS, 2002).

Exposure to psychic loads can trigger problems such as emotional exhaustion, mental imbalance, digestive disorders and migraines. This can affect the quality of care offered to patients and the quality of life of the worker (MININEL; BABTISTA; FELLI, 2011).

With regard to biological risk, this is defined as the probability of occupational exposure to biological agents such as microorganisms, whether genetically modified or not, cell cultures, parasites, toxins and prions. Thus, during occupational exposure to blood, at least 20 pathogens can be transmitted directly or indirectly, with the

Human Immunodeficiency Virus (HIV), Hepatitis B Virus (HBV) and Hepatitis C Virus (HCV) standing out for their greater epidemiological and clinical importance (ALMEIDA et al, 2009).

Nursing professionals are one of the categories working in the hospital environment who are most exposed to these risks; this is due to the fact that they are in direct contact with patients (MICHEL, 2000). Accidents involving sharps are very common, usually due to the lack of measures to prevent and control this type of accident (MARZIALE, 2002).

Exposure to these biological agents is most often caused by the daily handling of contaminated sharps, due to the need to manipulate needles, intravenous catheters, blades and other materials to carry out technical nursing procedures. Interest in the occupational exposure of health workers to pathogens, especially blood-borne pathogens, arose from the HIV/AIDS epidemic in the 80s. In order to protect these professionals, occupational safety and health measures were implemented, in particular the so-called Universal Precautions (PU), established in 1996 by the *Center for Disease Control and Prevention* (CDC) and Regulatory Standard No. 32 (NR32) - Safety and Health at Work in Health Services, established by the Ministry of Labor and Employment - Brazil (MTE), approved through Ordinance No. 485, of November 11, 2005. These rules should be used to assist all patients, regardless of their pathology, when handling blood, secretions, excretions, contact with mucous membranes and non-integrated skin (CANALLI; MORIYA; HAYASHIDA, 2011; MACHADO; MACHADO, 2011; ALVES; PASSOS; TOCANTINS, 2009; SOARES et al, 2012).

According to Chiodi, Marziale and Robazzi (2007), biological agents are present in exposure to blood and bodily fluids that cause infections; pathogens are transmitted by blood such as hepatitis B (HBV), hepatitis C (HCV), Acquired Immunodeficiency Syndrome (AIDS), which can be fatal. Contamination usually occurs via the skin, caused by accidents at work with sharp material.

The occupational risks identified among nursing professionals, especially biological risks, are greater when they are related to the direct care provided to patients and the characteristics of patients, such as critically ill patients (NISHIDE; BENATTI, 2004).

It is worth noting that the identification of occupational risks has a preventive nature in terms of work-related illnesses and accidents. It is important for nursing professionals to have knowledge of occupational health, since they can act as agents for preventing and promoting their own health and that of the team (LEITAO; FERNANDES; RAMOS, 2008).

It is believed that nursing workers are aware of some of the occupational risks present in the workplace. However, they associate these risks with the profession, and still consider exhausting dedication as part of the vocation to practice nursing. This is one of the main reasons why professionals omit to report accidents at work, which is detrimental to their investigation and prevention (LEITAO; FERNANDES; RAMOS, 2008).

In view of this, it is important to know and understand the definition of occupational accidents suffered by nursing professionals, since they are exposed to occupational risk factors and consequently to the occurrence of such accidents.

CHAPTER 3

Accidents at work among nursing staff

With the changes that have taken place in the world of work, as well as the increased demands on working environments, there has also been an increase in the psychological overload on workers, which can often not promote healthy living and working conditions. As a result, over the years, the number of records of accidents and work-related illnesses has grown, generating an impact on the rates of illnesses related to psychological disorders (KAMIMURA; TAVARES, 2012).

The impact of globalization on work production, demands for professional qualifications, competitiveness and threats of job cuts have had a number of effects on workers' mental health (FLACH et al., 2009). According to the WHO, the demands arising from globalization are factors that can contribute to the growth of accidents at work and incidences of work-related illnesses. The WHO also states that work-related accidents and illnesses cause the deaths of 1.1 million people worldwide every year (WHO, 1999).

According to data from the Ministry of Social Security (MPS), there has been a slight reduction in the occurrence of reported accidents at work in Brazil. This was evident when comparing the incidence of these accidents in 2010, 2011 and 2012. It is worth noting that in 2010 there were 709,474 cases of accidents at work; in 2011 there were 720,629 cases; and in 2012 there were fewer than in 2011 and 2010, with 705,239 cases, according to the National Classification of Economic Activities (CNAE) (BRASIL, 2012).

Brazil is the fourth nation in the world with the most accidents at work, behind only China, India and Indonesia. Since 2012, the economy has suffered an impact of R$22 billion due to people taking time off work after suffering injuries at work. If accidents in informal occupations were included, this figure could reach R$40 billion (CORREIO BRAZILIENSE, 2017).

Based on this information, it can be seen that accidents at work represent serious public health and economic problems for a country. In many industrial sectors there has been a reduction in accidents at work, while in the health sector there has been an increase in these incidents, especially in hospital environments (RUIZ;

BARBOZA; SOLER, 2004).

For the Ministry of Social Security, accidents at work are those that occur in the course of work at the service of the company or in the course of work by insured persons, which can cause consequences such as bodily injury and/or functional disturbance. This can lead to permanent or temporary loss or impairment of the ability to work, or even death. In the case of nursing workers, among the various injuries that affect them are those caused by accidents at work and work-related illnesses (BRASIL, 2012; SECCO et al., 2010).

Also similar to accidents at work are accidents linked to work, those which occur at the insured person's place of work and during working hours, illnesses caused by accidental contamination by the worker in the course of their work, and accidents suffered by the worker in the service of the company or on the way from home to work or from work to home (BRASIL, 2012).

The main concepts related to accidents at work are classified as follows: accident with a Registered Accident Report (CAT) (corresponding to the number of accidents for which the CAT has been registered with the National Institute of Social Security (INSS)); accident without a registered CAT (corresponding to the number of accidents for which the CAT has not been registered with the INSS); typical accidents (accidents arising from the characteristics of the professional work carried out by the injured person); commuting accidents (accidents occurring on the way from home to work or from work to the insured person's home); accidents due to occupational diseases (accidents caused by some type of occupational disease typical of a particular line of work, listed in the Social Security table); liquidated accident (refers to the number of accidents with cases closed by the INSS after treatment has been completed and the sequelae have been compensated); medical assistance (corresponds to insured workers who have only received medical assistance for their recovery to work); temporary incapacity (refers to workers who are temporarily incapacitated for work); permanent incapacity (refers to insured workers who remain permanently incapacitated for work activities, and the incapacity can be partial or total); and death (corresponds to the number of insured workers who died as a result of the accident at work) (BRASIL, 2012).

According to a survey carried out by the Ministry of Social Security in 2012, the number of accidents at work with a CAT recorded was 541,286, of which 423,935 were typical accidents at work, 102,396 were commuting accidents and 14,955 were classified as accidents due to occupational diseases. It also found a total of 163,953 accidents at work without a registered CAT (BRASIL, 2012).

When it comes to restoring the health of injured workers, it can be seen that the structure offered by the government is precarious. This is because the quality of medical care is hampered by limited financial resources and also because the Unified Health System (SUS) offers care with limited resources to the entire population, along with care for workers injured at work (ROCHA, 2002).

It should be noted that accidents at work can and must be prevented. These accidents can have a major impact on the economy and productivity, and can also cause great social suffering. It is estimated that occupational diseases and illnesses cause a loss of 4% of the Gross Domestic Product (GDP) in developed countries, and 10% in developing countries such as Brazil (SANTANA et al., 2006).

In the context of the theme "accidents at work and nursing", it should be noted that in most hospital and non-hospital environments, work is risky and unhealthy, so that workers perform their tasks in inadequate ways. Often, these professionals do not use protective equipment correctly or the physical structure is inappropriate, and there are no suitable working conditions in the establishment. These factors can compromise the individual's work practice and quality of life in their working environment, leaving them susceptible to accidents. This contradicts Regulatory Standard (NR) No. 32, drawn up by the Brazilian Ministry of Labor and Employment (ROBAZZI; BARROS JUNIOR, 2005).

These hospital nursing professionals are exposed to accidents of various kinds resulting from their work activities (SECCO et al., 2010). This is due to the fact that these professionals are subject to various occupational risk factors, as mentioned above. One reality is that even though they have a concept of the profession, professionals often do not attribute the accidents and illnesses they suffer at work as being due to their work activities (ROBAZZI; MARZIALE, 1999).

Some research has shown a higher frequency of occupational accidents among nursing professionals when compared to other healthcare workers (BAKKEA; ARAUJO, 2010; VELASCO et al., 2014). Nursing staff are the most exposed to accidents at work. Accidents involving this type of worker account for 73.6% of all occurrences. This factor highlights the concern for the health of these professionals, since they are subject to occupational risks due to the particularities of the care they provide to patients directly and uninterruptedly (BAKKEA; ARAUJO, 2010). In many cases, this factor can be justified by the fact that the institution does not have an effective policy to promote safety at work. This leads to unsafe conditions and a lack of assistance for the injured professional.

Benatti (1997) found in his study that, in a population of hospital nursing workers, the lack of time for leisure is an important factor that exposes workers to the risk of accidents. This is due to professionals adopting tiring and strenuous postures in their work activities. Gelbcke (1991) states that living conditions, relationships and the work process itself are basic conditioning factors for the health and illness process of nursing professionals.

In this sense, these characteristics become important, as the work of the nursing team is mainly focused on the administration of medication, which involves the constant handling of needles, scalpels and other sharp devices. In view of this, it is important that these activities are carried out with attention and care, given that any carelessness on the part of the professional can lead to an accident (GIR et al., 2008; VALIM; MARZIALE, 2011).

According to Valim and Marziale (2011), the main factors favoring accidents with sharp objects are linked to the working conditions in which professionals carry out their activities, especially unhealthy conditions and hazards. This is due to the lack of adequate working conditions, such as the disposal of material in inappropriate places and the lack of safety equipment.

Still in this context of drug administration, Leitao, Fernandes and Ramos (2008) report that nursing staff are exposed to the risk of drug absorption on a daily basis, when they handle drugs without the use of appropriate equipment, characterizing the chemical risk. Souto (2005) states that approximately 5% of nursing professionals become sensitive to antibiotics when they are handled incorrectly. He also states that some immunosuppressant drugs can cause teratogenic and carcinogenic reactions. These reports show how vulnerable nursing staff are to occupational risks, both in the administration and preparation of medicines, exposing professionals to the risk of accidents.

Accidents can also be related to the socio-economic difficulties that workers face due to the devaluation of their activities and unsatisfactory pay. Professionals may feel obliged to adjust their schedules to take on exhausting working hours (SECCO et al., 2010).

For the Federal Nursing Council (COFEN), double formal employment is an indicator related to the working conditions of nurses. It refers to the fact that approximately 70% of professionals work under these conditions, which can favor the occurrence of accidents at work (BRASIL, 1995).

In light of the above, it should be borne in mind that a profession such as nursing has difficulties in terms of professional appreciation. This factor can interfere with professionals' self-esteem, as it subjects them to numerous factors that make accidents at work even more damaging for these workers (SECCO et al., 2010).

With regard to the causes and reasons that can lead to accidents, studies show a variety of factors that contribute to these occurrences. Of these factors, the speed of tasks, lack of attention during the execution of a procedure, physical and mental fatigue of the worker, work overload, lack of experience of the professional, absence of Personal Protective Equipment (PPE), agitation of the patient during care, inadequate procedure, lack of team contribution and excessive self-confidence are among the most reported in research (DAMACENO et al., 2006; SILVA NETO; ALEXANDRE; SOUSA, 2014; SIMAO et al., 2010). It is worth mentioning that these situations expose workers to occupational stress, leaving them vulnerable to accidents at work.

According to Appolinario (2008), nursing professionals are more likely to suffer from hypertension, orthopedic diseases, diabetes *mellitus,* neurological disorders and other illnesses. This is justified by the overload of work and the psychic suffering of professionals, due to economic difficulties and double working hours. It should be noted that some of these pathologies may be related to and triggered by the work the worker does, which may vary according to the sector in which they work.

In this context, it should be noted that some hospital sectors may present more occupational risks than others, which may vary according to the activities carried out by the professionals and the severity of the patients and their pathologies. It is therefore possible to state that the risks that workers are exposed to are inherent to the procedures and complexity of the care provided in the sector where they work (BAKKEA; ARAUJO, 2010).

Cunha, Queiroz and Tavares (2009) state that the need for speed in procedures, the low quality of safety equipment and the lack of training for professionals, due to turnover between sectors, are frequent reasons why accidents occur. With this in mind, they mention that NR 32 obliges the permanent training of professionals through continuing education. This is especially important when the professional is transferred to another sector, since they are exposed to occupational risks that are different from those in their original sector.

Lima, Pinheiro and Viera (2007) state that the routine of nursing staff in hospital environments is permeated by tiredness, stress, haste, inattention and overload. This favors the occurrence of accidents at work, since attention, concentration and care during activities can prevent errors in the course of care.

In view of the above, it can be seen that nursing aids need to be improved and standardized in institutions, in order to use safety cultures, accident prevention and biosafety measures in the work of these professionals. In this way, accidents can be avoided or minimized, depending on the team's adherence to the standard measures, as well as their concentration, attention and care when carrying out their tasks (ALMEIDA; BENATTI, 2010).

It is also worth mentioning that the working environment of nursing professionals can be harmful to their health. This is due to unfavorable conditions for professional satisfaction and quality of life, caused by excessive physical and mental activity. As a result, it is clear that nursing work can be precarious, and that these factors determine the occurrence of accidents and occupational illnesses (GIOMO et al., 2009; MAURO; VEIGA, 2008).

As a result, when workers develop an occupational illness or are involved in accidents, they may be absent from work. This factor confirms that nursing professionals go through various processes of wear and tear, generating damage that compromises the worker's quality of life throughout their lives (SANTANA et al., 2013). These accidents and illnesses increase the incidence of absenteeism among nursing staff. This can lead to an overload of work for other members of the nursing team, hindering the development of activities aimed at service users.

It is therefore possible to conclude that nursing workers are exposed to various occupational risks, even without suffering any kind of accident. It is therefore up to hospital managers to adopt measures to promote and prevent the health of these workers, since they will always be exposed to such risks due to the need to carry out their care and administrative activities.

Based on this context, there is a need for nursing workers to be informed about the occupational risks present in the environment in which they work, which can cause them physical and/or mental exhaustion. It is therefore up to managers to promote the health of workers in the hospital environment, through courses, continuing education and psychosocial support, in order to provide them with better working conditions and quality of life, which results in a better quality of care.

23

CHAPTER 4

Self-esteem and nursing

Emotional problems can affect individuals due to friction with their work organization. In this sense, they can generate illnesses that are defined as psychosomatic (RANGEL, 2009). According to the Ministry of Health's Manual of Procedures for Health Services, disappointments at work, accumulated *deficits* due to long years of work, loss of job and dismissal are occupational risk factors and are related to changes in self-esteem (BRASIL, 2001).

According to Gallar (1998), self-esteem is related to a person's personality, which can result from who the individual is, how they perceive things and how others perceive them, influencing their self-worth and confidence in their relationships.

Considerations of self-esteem and self-concept, as well as the personal dimensions of being, having, being able and wanting, are fundamental to people's coexistence. Thus, according to Gomes (1997), the individual's construction of their self-concept is made possible by self-esteem, through cognitive capacity and modes of conduct and performance, followed by special attitudes towards them (PLACCO, 2001).

Self-esteem is designated by confidence, by the human capacity to think, by the right to win and be happy, by the ability to face life's challenges. The essence of self-esteem is related to the confidence of one's own ideas and the awareness of being worthy of happiness. This confidence becomes a motivational and behavioral factor. Thus, it is believed that the level of self-esteem can influence acts and ways of acting (BRANDEN, 2000).

Self-esteem can also be considered as a set of beliefs that one has and accepts as true in relation to one's self, one's competence and what one can do. Thus, it includes the confidence to think about and face life's challenges, the will to grow and be happy, individual integrity, the feeling of being deserving, worthy, considered capable of expressing one's needs and desires, in order to enjoy the results of due effort (SABBI, 1999).

With this, the definition of self-esteem suggests the commitment of the human being in their awareness of the possibilities of choice, and feeling free at a moment's notice to exercise their power of decision. It is also a characteristic of the individual who, at certain moments, experiences an intimate willingness to practice the capacities of their own consciousness (BRANDEN, 1995; 2000). For Rosenberg (1965), self-esteem is a judgment that the individual makes and usually keeps about himself, expressing attitudes of approval or disapproval.

Self-esteem theories have been described by various authors. Table 1 shows some of the theorists who describe definitions, approaches and limitations of self-esteem.

Chart 1 - Self-esteem theories according to authors.

Author	Definition	Approach	Limitations
Robert White	An evolutionary phenomenon, self-esteem is linked to concepts of competence and ego effectiveness.	Psychodynamics	Based on theoretical assumptions of structures of the personality and it can't be experimentally evaluated
William James	Relation to values, competence and success for each individual	It is based on historical perspective	It is based on introspection
Morris Rosenberg	Positive or negative attitude towards a particular object, the "self". Self-efficacy and value	Sociocultural	Self-esteem depends on the environment, i.e. personal motivation is undervalued from this point of view
Nathaniel Branden	Four pillars support the self-esteem: integrity as a person, degree of awareness, self-acceptance and willingness to accept responsibility	Humanist	More work philosophical that scientific. Aimed at laypeople looking for self-help reading
Seymor Epstein	Hierarchical structure which is based on cognitive organization	Cognitive-experimental	The personality development than self-esteem

Stanley Coopersmith	Self-esteem depends on experience and behavior. Learning is the key word	Behavioral	Most studies have been restricted to childhood and adolescence

Source: (TERRA, 2010; ROCHA, 2002).

It is worth noting that this construct reflects positive or negative attitudes towards the individual. Thus, it is considered a set of feelings and thoughts about one's own value, competence and adequacy (ROSENBERG, 1965). The main point of self-esteem is the evaluative aspect and this is because it influences how the individual chooses their goals, accepts themselves, appreciates others and outlines their expectations for the future (COOPERSMITH, 1989).

According to Vargas, Dantas and Gois (2005), self-esteem can be classified as high or low. When it is high, the individual expresses feelings that they think they are good enough. When low, the individual feels self-rejection, dissatisfaction and contempt for themselves. The level of acceptance or rejection of the *self* covers the whole of the individual's life, since it is a learning phenomenon. Branden (2000) assesses self-esteem according to low, medium and high levels. Low self-esteem is measured by a feeling of incompetence, nonconformity with life and an inability to overcome challenges. High self-esteem is assessed by the expression of feelings of competence and confidence and medium self-esteem manifests an inconsistency in behavior that fluctuates between feelings of adaptation or inadequacy.

It should also be noted that high self-esteem correlates with rationality, intuition, realism, independence, creativity, flexibility, the ability to accept change, the willingness to accept and correct mistakes, cooperation and benevolence. However, low self-esteem correlates with irrationality, rigidity, blindness to reality, fear of the new, rebelliousness, a defensive posture and fear of hostility towards oneself (BRANDEN, 2000).

Individuals with high self-esteem maintain an image of their abilities and their distinctiveness as a person. These individuals are also more likely to take active roles in social groups (COOPERSMITH, 1967). Individuals who are motivated to have high self-esteem have signs of a positive self-concept, which can be developed through each person's life experiences. This element of self-concept is determined as a set of personal thoughts and feelings, which have the individual themselves as a referential object (ROSENBERG, 2014).

When self-esteem is high, the individual feels confident, competent, valued, can cope with challenges and easily adapts to life's events. When self-esteem is medium, the person fluctuates between right and wrong, appropriate and inappropriate. When self-esteem is low, the individual always feels wrong, sensitive to criticism, inferior, isolated, insecure and conformed. In this way, it is understood that the higher a worker's level of self-esteem, the better he or she will cope with adversity, thus obtaining better chances of success and healthy relationships (BRANDEN, 2000; TERRA, 2010).

Still in this context, it is worth pointing out that nursing workers, like any human being, face difficult situations, professional devaluation, explosive moments and despair. However, when they have high self-esteem, they can quickly recover their normal state. This is because they consider these adversities to be momentary shocks, which are not capable of affecting people with a high level of satisfaction (QUIALA; RODRIGUEZ, 1999).

Individuals with low self-esteem can experience problems such as family violence, early pregnancy, drug abuse, poor school performance, school aggression, suicide, delinquency, depression and prostitution (ASSIS; AVANCI, 2003; DOURADO, 1984; GOMES, 1994; ROSENBERG, 1989; MECCA; SMELSER; VASCONCELLOS, 1989; TAMAYO; CUNHA, 1983).

A survey of nursing staff found that 24.4% of them had psychiatric illnesses, with depression being the most common (VIEIRA et al., 2013). Therefore, it is noteworthy that people with low self-esteem are 39 times more likely to have depressive symptoms when compared to people with high self-esteem (HALL et al., 1996).

Low self-esteem can severely limit an individual's inspirations and achievements. Its consequences can be presented indirectly, like a "ticking time bomb", which silently pushes the individual to demonstrate their abilities without a real need. In this way, the person starts working without due care, which leads them to make mistakes and cause unhappiness in their work and personal life, as well as accidents at work (BRANDEN, 2011).

It should be noted that self-esteem can be influenced by factors such as gender, marital status, age and the presence of certain pathologies. There are signs that demonstrate an individual's self-esteem. These can be physical, psychological and emotional, such as: a balanced posture, self-acceptance, self-love, security, trust in other people, self-confidence, among others (LEE; SHEHAN, 1989; SCHIEMAN;

CAMPBELL, 2001; SABBI, 1999).

The study by Cooper and Dewe (2008) carried out in 2006 and 2007 showed that work-related illnesses were responsible for approximately 30 million days lost from work. Of these, 13.8 million days lost were due to stress, depression or anxiety, highlighting that these conditions can alter an individual's self-esteem.

Also in this context, the aim of meeting basic needs is associated with levels of psychological health. Therefore, workers who have the respect and admiration of co-workers, managers and family members can develop their self-esteem better, progressively favoring psychological balance. It is therefore believed that self-esteem is directly related to favorable work performance (MASLOW, 1954).

CHAPTER 5

Stress and nursing

The term stress is part of the vocabulary of the average citizen. We hear about it not only in everyday conversations, but also on television, radio and in newspapers. The number of conferences, courses and researchers in this field has multiplied. However, sometimes, when we cross-reference these different types of information, their meaning is unclear. The meaning given to the word *stress* acquires different meanings both at the explanatory level, as a theoretical construct, and at the level of experimental research (MENDES, 2002).

Stress has been investigated along three main lines: the biological response it causes (from aspects of the central nervous system to its vegetative, endocrine, immune and general behavioral repercussions), the events that trigger it and the transition that is established between the individual and the environment in these circumstances. Regardless of these points of view, it is important to consider the importance of social support as a mitigating factor in the impact of stress-inducing circumstances on the individual (SERRA, 2002).

The first references to the word stress meaning affliction and adversity date back to the 14th century (LAZARUS; FOLKMAN, 1994), but its use was sporadic and non-systematic. In the 17th century, the word, which originates from the Latin *stringere,* came to be used in English to designate oppression, discomfort and adversity (SPIELBERGER, 1979 apud LIPP, 1996).

In 1932, Walter B. Cannon, in his book The Wisdom of the Body, used the term "emergency reaction" to describe how human beings who react inadequately to the psychic demands of their living environment, being psychologically unprepared, can develop abnormal wear and tear on their organism and present a chronic inability to tolerate, overcome or adapt, presenting injuries ranging from restlessness to exhaustion or mental dullness, depending on their psychic structure (VIEIRA; SCHULLER SOBRINHO,
1995) .

Later, in 1936, endocrinologist Hans Selye introduced the term stress to designate a syndrome produced by various harmful agents. His focus was on the organism's non-specific response to situations that weakened it or made it ill, which he called the General Adaptation Syndrome or Biological Stress Syndrome, also commonly known as the syndrome of simply being ill (LAZARUS; FOLKMAN, 1994).

This endocrinologist was responsible for the first experimental evidence of stress, conducted at McGill University in Canada. Looking for new hormones in the placenta, he injected a placental extract intraperitoneally into rats and found a series of changes. These, however, could not be attributed to the effects of this extract, since the control animals, injected with placebo, had the same changes. Selye suggested the hypothesis that manipulation and/or injection could be responsible for the changes found. To test this hypothesis, he exposed the animals to a series of different stimuli, including cold, tissue injury, excessive exercise and intoxication, and observed the same findings regardless of the stimulus used. He concluded that it was a general alarm reaction to critical situations and that it represented an effort by the body to adapt to the new condition, and then called it General Adaptation Syndrome (GAS). This syndrome was characterized by hypertrophy of the adrenal glands, gastric ulcers and a decrease in the size of the thymus, bony and lymphatic ganglia (SELYE, 1936).

Selye's work was greatly influenced by the discoveries of two physiologists who made an impact at the time: Bernard, who in 1879 had suggested that the internal environment of organisms should remain constant despite changes in the external environment, and Cannon, who in 1939 suggested the name homeostasis to designate the effort of physiological processes to maintain the state of internal balance in the organism. Selye, using these concepts, defined stress as a breakdown in this balance (LIPP, 1996).

In fact, the term stress was used with the connotation it has today: it is the way in which the body responds to any stimulus - good, bad, evil or imaginary - that alters its state of equilibrium. It is directly related to homeostasis, which is the state of balance between the various systems of the organism and between the organism as a whole and the environment. The concept of stress sees it as a bio-psycho-social process, because of the way it manifests itself, dependent on individual characteristics and the social environment (SELYE, 1956).

The body's reactions to the pressures exerted by the situations experienced give rise to stress, which is the sum of the body's unspecific changes in response to a stimulus or situation. SAG has been described, which can be understood as the set of all the general reactions of the body that accompany prolonged exposure to a stressor and comprises three phases: alert or alarm reaction - tachycardia, paleness, fatigue, insomnia, lack of appetite, chest pressure, tense stomach; resistance or adaptive reaction - social isolation, inability to disconnect from work, impotence for activities, heaviness in the shoulders; and exhaustion - depression (SELYE, 1956).

Stress is a reaction of the organism, with physical and/or psychological components, caused by the psychophysiological changes that occur when a person is confronted with a situation that, in one way or another, irritates, frightens, excites, confuses or even makes them immensely happy (LIPP,
1996) .

It is a set of reactions of the organism to physical, psychological, infectious and other aggressions capable of disturbing its homeostasis (DELBONI,
1997) . It is one of the constructs widely studied by sports psychology, due to its consequences for performance (LIPP, 1996), and is understood by Samulski (2002) as the product of man's relationship with the physical and socio-cultural environment. It represents a complex process of the organism, interrelating biochemical, physical and psychological aspects, triggered by the way stimuli are processed (REINHOLD, 2011). Emotional and physical tension, constantly felt, leads to a state of stress, which, like most syndromes, does not occur overnight, but builds up slowly (DELBONI, 1997).

Stress is a substantial imbalance between physical and/or psychological demand and the ability to respond, under conditions in which failure to meet that demand results in consequences. The stress process consists of four interrelated stages, which are described as follows: the first is the environmental demand, i.e. when some kind of demand is imposed on the individual; the second is the perception of the demand, which can be explained as the different ways in which situations are perceived, whether threatening or not; The third stage is the response to stress, which involves physical and psychological reactions to the perception of the situation, which can be changes in the level of activation, anxiety, muscle tension and changes in attention; and finally, in the fourth stage, behavioral consequences arise, which in this case refer to performance and results (McGRATH, 1970).

The positive level of stress was defined by Selye as *eustress*. However, if situations, good or bad, recur frequently, i.e. are constant, then there is a big problem. This negative process, characterized by distressing situations, is called *distress,* which can be acute (when it is intense, but for a short period, such as the news of the death of a loved one) or chronic (when it is not so intense, but has occurred repeatedly or constantly, such as tense situations in the workplace; worrying about debts that you don't know how to pay or repeated training without adequate intervals for the body to recover) (FIAMONCINI; FIAMONCINI, 2003).

It's true that stress is associated with many negative aspects, but this doesn't mean that it is in itself something to be removed from life at any time and in any way. Like salt, in the right quantities and conditions, stress is not only not bad, but it is necessary and can be decisive, or at least very important, for a satisfactory life. Excessive stress, like salt, can be unpleasant or biologically harmful (LABRADOR, 1992).

Situations experienced as stressful have an influence on the modification of individuals' immune responses. Personal variables such as coping strategies and *locus of* control have also been shown to mediate these influences (MENDES, 2002).

In the context of work, occupational stress is focused on organizational stressors, which can be differentiated by two types of stress-related studies: occupational stress and general stress. The former emphasize stressors related to the work environment and the latter, general stressors in the individual's life (SCHMIDT, 2009).

Stress related to the work environment has been widely studied in recent decades, under different approaches, in order to identify its role in the etiology of health alterations in workers (ARAUJO et al., 2003; JUAREZ-GARCIA, 2007). This can perhaps be explained by the fact that the working environment has changed and kept pace with advances in technology more quickly than the ability of workers to adapt, who now live under continuous tension, not only in the workplace, but in life in general.

The type of wear and tear that people are permanently subjected to in their work environments and relationships are determining factors of illness. Psychosocial stressors are as powerful as microorganisms and unhealthy conditions in triggering illness. Both workers and executives can show changes in the face of psychosocial stressors (BALLONE, 2011).

The emotional strain found in relationships with work is a very significant factor in determining stress-related disorders, such as depression, pathological anxiety, panic, phobias, psychosomatic illnesses, among others. In short, people with this type of occupational stress do not respond to the demands of the job and are generally irritable and depressed (CARNEIRO, 2011).

One of the aggravating factors of work-related stress is the limitation to which society subjects individuals when it comes to expressing their anxieties, frustrations and emotions. Because of social norms and rules, people end up being prisoners of political correctness, obliged to show emotional or motor behavior that is incongruous with their real feelings of aggression or fear (CARNEIRO, 2011).

There are many stressful stimuli in the workplace. Significant anxiety (alarm reaction) can be experienced in the face of disagreements with colleagues, overload and the race against time, salary dissatisfaction and, depending on the person, even the ringing of the telephone. Disorganization in the workplace puts order and the worker's ability to perform at risk. Generally, conditions worsen when there is a lack of clarity in the rules, regulations and tasks that each worker must perform, as well as in unhealthy environments, with a lack of suitable tools, among others (BALLONE, 2011).

In recent years, there has been a growing interest in the study of stress and work-related psychosocial factors, due to the repercussions they can have on workers' health. Occupational stress is not a new phenomenon, but a recent field of study that has been emphasized due to the emergence of diseases that have been linked to work-related stress, such as hypertension, gastric ulcers and others (STACCIARINI; TROCOLLI, 2000).

Stress has consequences for health and quality of life. These can be seen in sick leave, a drop in productivity and interpersonal difficulties, generating high personal and professional costs. It is necessary to identify sources of stress in organizations, which interfere with individual well-being and performance (SADIR; LIPP, 2009).

These psychosocial factors can lead to the phenomenon called presenteeism, in which people are present at their jobs, but due to problems such as health problems, they are unable to carry out their tasks (NOBEN et al., 2014). The worker is present even though their state of health is poor and they have a certain fragility to justify their absence from work (KRANE et al., 2014). Their productivity is reduced or unsatisfactory and may be related to their health conditions; this reduction causes damage and harm to all those involved in the work process and the end result of the service (WADA et al., 2013).

The stressors of the work environment have also caused an increase in cases of Burnout Syndrome in workers from different areas. Burnout Syndrome (BS) or "Professional Burnout" is a psychological syndrome resulting from the chronic emotional tension experienced by the worker, characterized by emotional exhaustion, depersonalization and low personal accomplishment that can affect professionals whose work requires direct contact with the public, especially when it involves care and assistance activities, (TIRONI et al., 2009).

BS is recognized worldwide as one of the major psychosocial problems affecting the quality of life of professionals in various fields, especially those involving health care, education and human services, and is directly involved in the stressors of the work environment (SOUSA; MEDONQA, 2009).

The International Labor Organization (ILO) defines work-related stress as a set of phenomena that occur in workers' bodies and can affect their health. The main stress-generating factors present in the work environment involve aspects of the organization, management and work system and the quality of human relations (ILO, 1986).

More and more emphasis is being placed on the prophylaxis of excessive stress, including socio-psychological factors such as the suitability of the occupation or task for the human being (CRANDALL; PERREWE, 1995), human re-engineering (ZEITLIN, 1995), factors linked to ergometry and the work environment and also variables related to the stages of human life, such as pregnancy, childhood, adolescence, adulthood and ageing. The implications of stress for human productivity are addressed, as are the effects of political and social changes, which are stressors that affect the health and longevity of populations (LIPP, 1996).

In the health sector, working in unhealthy environments can obviously pose risks to workers' health, including the presence of physical and mental stress. Working conditions and environments consist of a set of variables which, directly or indirectly, can have an impact on life and health; this influence will depend on the individual's ability to adapt and resist risk factors. These variables, including the content and organization of work, the duration and configuration of working time, the remuneration system, opportunities to participate in improving these conditions, among other factors, can influence the physical, mental and social conditions of workers (ROBAZZI; MARZIALE, 1999).

The health-disease process does not happen in a linear fashion, but dynamically. This means that it will have the character of a spiral that alternately and permanently moves from health to illness. The modes of production trigger individual psycho-emotional processes that actually become manifestations of a collective. However, the manifestation of an individual symptom can be an indication that it is not just one individual who is getting sick, but the expression of a larger group that is sick in the organization (EGRY, 1996).

Concern about suffering and pleasure in the work of nursing professionals arose from questions about how these professionals managed to endure such exhausting work, especially because they had to live with suffering, pain and death so frequently (SHIMIZU; CIAMPONE, 1999).

Out of fear of the consequences of a mistake for themselves and the patient, they internalize control over their work excessively. This mechanism can lead them to develop a kind of paranoid proneness, i.e. the internalization of persecutory feelings in the absence of a concrete persecutor. This mechanism is adopted unconsciously by nurses as a way of protecting themselves from the unpredictability of its consequences, since, in everyday life, absolute control over their work is almost impossible, and they are often threatened by the possibility of mistakes. In order to avoid loss of control, feelings of guilt and punishment, these professionals become vigilant of themselves, attentive controllers of the results of their actions and experience fear of the consequences of an inattentive attitude (HOGA, 2002).

Occupational stress is determined by the worker's perception of the demands at work and their ability to cope with them. Hence the importance of learning more about this type of stress in order to develop strategies for dealing effectively with the problems it causes (STUMM, 2000).

CHAPTER 6

Self-esteem, stress and accidents at work among
nursing professionals

Work activities contribute to psychic alterations in nursing workers through various aspects. These include the complexity of factors related to work organization, such as the division of tasks, the organizational hierarchy and its management policies, the valuation and motivation of workers, among others. As a result, it can be said that mental and behavioral disorders related to the work of professionals are not the result of isolated factors alone, but of the work context and the interaction of the body with the psychic factor of the worker (BRASIL, 2001).

According to Batista et al. (2005), when it comes to motivating nurses, there is a considerable rise in the hierarchy of needs. In this way, the need for self-esteem among nursing professionals is lower than that of other professionals, showing that institutions have not valued the professional nurse, as well as the entire nursing team, for their qualities. As a result, the team does not receive the return for their activities performed with excellence, which reduces the level of self-esteem, and puts them in a zone of occupational risks or suffering at work, which can lead them to accidents at work, and an increase in stress levels.

The financial difficulties faced by many nursing workers are among the most common causes of distress, suffering and professional devaluation. Many of them even feel penalized by the lack of a salary increase. This factor is generated by the insecurity that the professional feels due to the fear of losing their job, and this contributes to them being subjected to precarious work regimes in unhealthy environments and with low salaries (ELIAS; NAVARRO, 2006; SECCO et al., 2010).

Insufficient pay can lead to the worker having to maintain another employment relationship, making it necessary to reconcile work activities in different shifts. In this way, they sacrifice their leisure and rest time to keep the other job. These factors can overburden nursing staff in their work activities, which leads to physical, psychological and social problems for their health (MAURO et al., 2010).

Adequate financial remuneration is a significant factor in motivating people to work in order to promote satisfaction, quality of life and professional development. In this sense, when wages are in line with work activities, they have a different denotation. This is due to the fact that it recognizes and values the activities carried out by the worker, which can raise their self-esteem and self-confidence, reducing levels of suffering and stress at work (NEVES et al., 2010).

It is therefore important for hospital institutions to maintain decent salaries, thus promoting satisfactory health and working conditions for workers. This is relevant in the sense that it increases their self-confidence, due to their recognition at work, and promotes better working and care conditions, free from suffering at work.

The occurrence of accidents at work can also be another factor of psychic suffering for nursing workers, which is another unfavorable point in terms of altered self-esteem. This is due to the professional's fear of falling ill as a result of the exposure caused by the accident, as well as the repercussions for their family and work colleagues. They are also embarrassed to have suffered the accident and to be judged as careless and incompetent. In this way, it can be seen that there are several factors that make accidents at work even more oppressive for nursing workers, enabling the manifestation of mental disorders, highlighting changes in levels of self-esteem (SECCO et al., 2010).

It is also worth emphasizing that the exposure of this team to biological materials caused by accidents has also been a factor in their suffering at work. In addition to facing emotional difficulties, such as stress, these workers are also subject to embarrassment for having suffered the accident. These factors can trigger problems with personal and social repercussions, causing alterations in the worker's well-being and psychic marks that are difficult to identify (SECCO et al., 2010). These factors contribute to the underreporting of accidents at work among hospital nursing staff.

Lancman and Sznelwar (2004) state that there are various forms of suffering at work. Among other disorders, we can mention fear of accidents at work, fear of aggression from users, anguish at the inability to follow the cadences or limits imposed, suffering from continuous repetition and boredom, fear of domination and authority exercised by the hierarchy.

The most sadistic direction of suffering lies in the intellectual void that the worker is subjected to. This is because they take responsibility for their anguish, leading to a permanent perception of incapacity and powerlessness at work. Based on this, it is possible to infer that with suffering at work, including the occurrence of accidents at work and stressful situations, workers can develop a change in their self-esteem, putting the quality of care, patient safety and their own health at risk (DEJOURS, 1999).

In view of the above, it is important to adopt measures to combat the stressors and motivators of psychic illnesses and changes in the self-esteem of nursing workers. This is due to the need for these individuals to have satisfactory physical and mental health in order to exercise their profession and provide care. High self-esteem therefore needs to be part of these workers' lives, to enable them to cope with challenges and adapt spontaneously to the various situations experienced in their profession and personal lives.

In addition to what has already been discussed, in the work environment, nursing workers are also influenced by various social factors, such as distance from home, embarrassment in traffic, lack of childcare facilities for their children, the responsibilities of the job, poor relations between the work team, fear of dismissal or retirement, the company's economic situation, among others. As a result, and over time, these factors can cause mental disturbances, such as boredom, stress and a sense of fatigue, which results in low self-esteem (MAURO, 1993; MAURO et al., 2010; SANTANA et al., 2013).

In many situations, the working hours of nursing staff are exhausting and stressful, due to the demand from users and the lack of time for rest, without adequate energy replenishment for work. In addition, these professionals are required to be totally committed and dedicated during the course of their work. As a result, they are more likely to suffer emotional distress, resulting in the total or partial loss of physiological and psychic capacities over time (FRANQA; FERRARI, 2012; LAURELL; NORIEGA, 1989).

Based on this context, it is possible to observe that by experiencing aspects that favor emotional exhaustion, nursing workers may be more exposed to psychiatric illness, including changes in self-esteem and chronic stress. In addition, the length of time they have been working can influence their mental health and their work activities, which does not favor high self-esteem and the quality of care provided to users.

The various factors present every day in the lives of nursing professionals, which contribute to psychic burdens, have an impact on the quality of life of these workers. The burdens generated are innumerable, and relate to fast-paced and repetitive work, lack of team interaction, pressure from managers and other colleagues, physical and mental fatigue, exhausting shifts, tension in the face of stressful situations, among others. These situations wear down the professional, putting them in inappropriate mental health conditions for nursing practice (RIBEIRO; SHIMIZU, 2007; SECCO et al., 2010).

In the midst of these findings, it is worth mentioning that the degree of complexity of the nursing team's tasks, together with the responsibilities and technical-scientific concerns, can contribute to possible mental alterations in the professional. As a result, these workers may not be able to perform their tasks safely. This impairs their professional performance and exposes them to the risk of accidents in the workplace (SILVA; PINTO, 2012).

The daily stresses that workers are subjected to in hospital environments can lead to greater mental exhaustion. This can lead to memory failures and reduced concentration in their work activities, leaving them susceptible to errors and accidents, which directly contributes to their psychic suffering and lower self-esteem (SANTOS; OLIVEIRA; MOREIRA, 2006).

According to Secco et al. (2010), in addition to the stresses and strains of their work, nursing professionals are exposed to suffering and emotional exhaustion resulting from the death, anguish, pain and difficulties of patients. These factors can have harmful consequences for their mental and physical health, resulting in low levels of self-esteem.

Emotional distress related to a stressful work environment can also be a significant factor in mental disorders (FERRAREZE; FERREIRA; CARVALHO, 2006). The pathway between psychic burdens and wear and tear can be immediate and have long-term consequences. This is due to the impact that the worker's mental and emotional health can suffer from the psychological abuse generated by stressors, which compromise their well-being, rationality, physical health and self-esteem (MININEL; BABTISTA; FELLI, 2011).

In view of the above, it can be concluded that emotional exhaustion can affect both the worker and their family, as well as the company, due to the reduction in tolerance to work stressors. This tends to leave them unable to cope with conflicts at work, reducing their productivity and quality of life. In this way, it is believed that institutions have a fundamental role to play in promoting workers' mental health, through preventive actions and quality of life programs for workers, since, as professionals feel good and have high self-esteem, the institution consequently improves productivity and quality of care, as well as being less exposed to the occurrence of accidents at work (ALVES, 2011).

It should be noted that accidents at work can have a direct impact on the mental health of nursing professionals, and that psychic suffering can compromise their work activities and reduce their self-esteem. In this way, we can see the importance of caring for the mental health of nursing professionals and promoting safety measures aimed at preventing accidents and work-related illnesses from occurring in the environments where they work. Therefore, it can be said that professionals will have adequate working conditions and a healthy life, which will consequently favor the quality of care provided to health service users.

FINAL CONSIDERATIONS

Nursing staff working in hospitals are exposed to various occupational risk factors that can compromise their physical and mental health. This exposure can leave them vulnerable to occupational accidents, stress at work and changes in self-esteem.

These workers often carry out their tasks in inadequate, stressful and repetitive conditions during the course of their working day, since this category is directly linked to the continuous and direct care of patients. This means that nursing professionals are exposed to occupational risks even if they don't suffer accidents in the workplace, due to the physical and mental strain caused by their work activities.

Therefore, there is a need to promote better working conditions in hospital environments. This is because it is necessary to promote a better quality of work and social life for nursing professionals.

It is worth noting that the psychic disorders experienced by nursing professionals at work, such as stress, also cause exposure to occupational risks; they can directly interfere with the self-esteem of these workers, which harms their quality of life and their work activities. This shows how important it is for nursing staff to maintain high self-esteem. This enables them to cope with the stressful situations of the profession and, consequently, promote better conditions for adapting to the various work and social situations.

In view of the above, it is essential to adopt measures to combat the stressors and motivators of psychiatric illness and altered self-esteem among nursing professionals, as these workers need to be in satisfactory physical and mental health in order to exercise their profession and provide care. To this end, high self-esteem needs to be an integral part of the daily lives of these professionals, favoring attention to the care provided to patients.

In this context, it is also suggested that measures be adopted to promote the quality of life and work of nursing professionals in hospital environments. These measures can be implemented through continuing education, to prevent the occurrence of accidents at work and factors that expose them to occupational risks; psychological support, to promote better mental conditions and counseling regarding work problems and stressors, reducing psychic suffering and emotional distress, as well as the incidence of chronic stress; physical activity in the workplace, to promote better physical conditions for workers and also to facilitate body and mental balance and coping strategies in the face of stressful situations in the daily lives of nursing professionals.

The identification of stressors at work can be considered an agent of change; once they have been identified, workers and managers can discuss them and propose possible solutions to minimize their effects, which can make the daily lives of nursing staff more productive, less stressful and make them more valued in terms of their human and professional aspects.

Occupational stress management programs should be designed and interventions planned to eliminate/minimize stressors in the workplace, including adjustments to the organizational structure, working conditions, training and personal development, participation and autonomy at work and interpersonal relationships. Interventions focused on the individual aim to reduce the impact of existing risks by developing an appropriate repertoire of individual coping strategies.

Some of the situations that lead to stress, such as work overload, lack of professional autonomy, continuous care for critically ill patients, lack of social support from superiors or family members, ineffective communication with colleagues, patients, patients' families and managers, difficulty in reconciling professional and family obligations, among others, will cease to exist if measures are taken at institutional and organizational level to encourage an improvement in the quality of information, starting with the training of workers and strengthening their social skills, including interpersonal relationships with patients, carers and colleagues.

In summary, we can see how important it is to take care of the mental health of nursing workers and to promote safety measures aimed at preventing work-related illnesses from occurring in hospital environments. Therefore, it can be said that professionals will have adequate working conditions and a healthier life, which will consequently favor the quality of care provided to health service users.

REFERENCES

ALMEIDA, C. A. F.; BENATTI, M. C. C. Occupational exposure of health care workers to organic fluids and adhesion to chemoprophylaxis. **Revista Escola de Enfermagem da USP** [Internet], v. 41, n. 1, p. 120-126, 2010. Available at: <http://www.scielo.br/pdf/reeusp/v41n1/v41n1a15.pdf>. Accessed on: Aug 17, 2015.

ALMEIDA, M. C. P. de. The construction of knowledge in nursing: historical evolution. In: NATIONAL SEMINAR ON NURSING RESEARCH. 1984, Florianopolis. **Proceedings...** Florianopolis, 1984. p. 58-77.

ALMEIDA, M. C. P.; ROCHA, J. S. Y. **O saber da enfermagem e sua dimensao pratica**. 2 ed. Sao Paulo, (SP): Cortez; 1989.

ALMEIDA, A. N. G.; et al. Biological risks among nursing workers. **Revista de Enfermagem da UERJ**, v. 17, n. 4, p. 595-600, 2009.

ALVES, E. F. Programs and support for quality of life at work. **Revista Interfacehs**, Sao Paulo, v.6, n.1, p. 60-78, Apr. 2011.

ALVES, S. S. M.; PASSOS, J. P.; TOCANTINS, F. R. Accidents with sharps in nursing workers: a question of biosafety. Revista de Enfermagem da UERJ, v. 17, n. 3, 373-377, 2009.

ANGERAMI, E.L.S.; CORREIA, F. de A. Em que consiste a enfermagem. **Revista da Escola de Enfermagem da USP,** Sao Paulo, v. 23, n. 3, p. 337-344, dec. 1989.

ANTUNES, J.L.F. **Hospital: institution and social history**. Sao Paulo: Letras & Letras, 1985.

APPOLINARIO, R. S. Absenteeism in the nursing team: analysis of scientific production. **Revista de Enfermagem da UERJ**, Rio de Janeiro, v. 16, n. 1, p. 83-87, jan./mar. 2008.

ARAUJO, T. M. et al. Aspectos psicossociais do trabalho e disturbios psiquicos entre trabalhadores de enfermagem. **Rev. Saude Publica,** Sao Paulo, v.37, n.4, p. 424-433, 2003.

ASSIS, S. G.; AVANCI, J. Q. **Labyrinth of mirrors.** The formation of self-esteem in childhood and adolescence. Rio de Janeiro, RJ: Editora Fiocruz, 2003.

BAKKEA, H. A.; ARAUJO, N. M. C. Accidents at work among health professionals at a university hospital. **Produpao**, Joao Pessoa, v. 20, n. 4, p. 669-676, Oct./Dec. 2010.

BALLONE, G. J. **Stress and Work**. Available at: <http://danielacarneiro.com/estresseetrabalho.aspx>. Accessed on: September 21, 2011.

BAPTISTA, R.C. Diseases and other health problems caused by work. **Cadernos**

interdisciplinares: saude, tecnologia e questao social, Rio de Janeiro, v. 1, n.1, p. 1-11,2004.

BARBOZA, J. I. R. A. et al. Evaluation of the sleep pattern of nursing professionals on night shifts in Intensive Care Units. **Einstein**, Sao Paulo, v.6, n.3, p. 296-301,2008.

BARRETO, M. M. S. **Violence, health and work:** a journey of humiliation. Sao Paulo: Educ, 2003.

BATISTA, A. A. V. et al. Factors of motivation and dissatisfaction in the work of nurses. **Revista da Escola de Enfermagem,** Sao Paulo, v. 39, n. 1, p. 85-91, 2005.

BELLATO, R.; PASTI, M. J.; TAKEDA, E. Algumas reflexoes sobre o metodo funcional no trabalho da enfermagem. **Revista Latino-Americana de Enfermagem,** Ribeirao Preto, v. 5, n. 1, p. 75-81, 1997.

BENATTI, M. C. C. **Occupational accidents in a university hospital**: a study on the occurrence and risk factors among nursing workers. Thesis [Doctorate]. USP Nursing School, Sao Paulo, 1997.

BEZERRA, A. M. F.; BEZERRA, K. K. S.; BEZERRA, W. K. T.; ATHAYDE, A. C. R.; VIEIRA, A. L. Occupational risks and work accidents in nursing professionals in the hospital environment. **REBES**, v. 5, n. 2, p. 01-07, 2015.

BORSOI, I. C. F.; CODO, W. Nursing, work and care. In: CODO, W.; SAMPAIO, J. J. C. **Sofrimento psiquico nas organizagoes**. Petropolis: Vozes, 1995.

BRANDEN, N. **Self-esteem and its pillars**. Sao Paulo: Saraiva, 1995.

. **Self-esteem:** how to learn to like yourself. Sao Paulo: Saraiva, 2000.

. **The power of self-esteem.** How to boost this important psychological resource. Barcelona, Paidos, 2011.

BRAZIL. Ministry of Labor and Employment. Regulatory Standard NR 9 - **Environmental Risk Prevention Program.** Portaria SSST n° 25, de 29 de dezembro de 1994. Brasilia, DF, 1994.

. Secretariat for Work Management and Health Education. Ministry of Health. **SIGTAP - Management system for work management.** Brasilia, 2010.

. Ministry of Health. **Work-related diseases: manual of procedures for health services**. Brasilia, 2001.

. Ministry of Health. **Workers' Health.** Brasilia, 2002 (Caderno de atengao basica, n. 5).

. Ministry of Social Security. **Statistical Yearbook of Accidents at Work**: 2013. Brasilia, 2013. Available at: <http://www.previdenciasocial.gov.br/arquivos/office>. Accessed: 12 Dec. 2015.

. Federal Nursing Council. **Resolution No. 186/95**. Rio de Janeiro, 1995.

. Federal Nursing Council. **Analysis of data on the registration of nursing professionals in the Regional Councils in 2011**. Brasilia, COFEN, 2013.

. Ministry of Health. National Network for Comprehensive Workers' Health Care. **Management Manual**. Sao Paulo, 2006.

. Ministry of Health. **Work-related diseases: manual of procedures for health services**. Brasilia, MS, 2001.

. Ministry of Social Security. **AEPS 2012 - Section IV - Accidents at Work**. Brasilia, 2012. Available at: <http://www.previdencia.gov.br/estatisticas/aeps-2012-secao-iv-acidentes-do- trabalho>. Accessed: May 12, 2014.

. CONSELHO REGIONAL DE ENFERMAGEM DE SAO PAULO. **Piso salarial das categorias de enfermagem**. Sao Paulo, 2007.

BRITO, A. A. F. B. The Fourth Industrial Revolution and the Prospects for Brazil. Revista Cientifica Multidisciplinar Nucleo do Conhecimento, ed. 07, v. 02, p. 91-96, 2017.

CAMELO, S. H. H.; ANGERAMI, E. L. S. Psychosocial risks related to the work of family health teams: professionals' perceptions. **Revista de Enfermagem da UERJ**, Rio de Janeiro, v. 15, n. 4, p. 502-507, Oct/Dec. 2007.

CAMPBELL, J.; MUPHY, L. R.; HURRELL, J. J. **Stress and wellbeing at work**. Washington: American Psychological Association, 1997.

CANALLI, R. T. C.; MORIYA, T. M.; HAYASHIDA, M. Prevention of accidents with biological material among nursing students. **Revista de Enfermagem da UERJ**, v. 19, n. 1, p. 100-106, 2011.

CARAN, V. C. S. **Psychosocial risks and bullying in the academic context**. 2007. 188 f. Dissertation (Master's in Nursing) - Ribeirao Preto School of Nursing, University of Sao Paulo, Ribeirao Preto, 2007.

CARNEIRO, D. **Stress and Work**. Available at: <http://danielacarneiro.com/estresseetrabalho.aspx>. Accessed on: September 26, 2011.

CHIODI, M. B.; MARZIALE, M. H. P.; ROBAZZI, M. L. C. C. Work accidents with biological material among workers in public health units. **Revista Latino-America de Enfermagem**, Ribeirao Preto, v.15, n. 4, p. 632-638, 2007.

COOPER, C.; DEWE, P. Well-being-absenteeism, presenteeism, costs and challenges. **Occupational Medicine**, Oxford ,v. 58, n. 8, p. 522-524, 2008.

COOPERSMITH, S. **The antecedents of self-esteem**. San Francisco: Freeman, 1967.

. Coopersmith Self-Esteem Inventory. **Consulting Psychologists Press**, Palo Alto,

1989.

CRANDALL, R.; PERREWE, P. **Occupational stress:** a handbook. New York: Taylor & Francis, 1995.

SOUZA, R. Accidents at work in Brazil. **Correio Braziliense**, 2017. Available at:http://www.correiobraziliense.com.br/app/noticia/economia/2017/06/05/internas_e conomia,600125/acidente-de-trabalho-no-brasil.shtml. Accessed: 06 Dec 2017.

CUNHA, A. C.; QUEIROZ, A. C.; TAVARES, C. M. M. Educapao continuada na prevenpao dos riscos biologicos da equipe de enfermagem de uma instituipao hospitalar. **Ciencia, Cuidado e Saude,** Maringa, v. 8, n. 3, p. 469-476, 2009.

DAMACENO, A. P. et al. Occupational accidents with biological material: the perception of the injured professional. **Revista Brasileira de Enfermagem**, Brasilia, v. 59, n. 1, p. 72-77, jan./feb. 2006.

DELBONI, T. H. **Overcoming Stress.** Sao Paulo: Makron Books, 1997.

DEJOURS, C. **The trivialization of social injustice**. Fundapao Getulio Vargas. Rio de Janeiro, 1999.

DOURADO, J. M. B. **O desempenho acadêmico e sua relapa com o autoconceito do aluno e a retroalimentação do professor**. Dissertation (Master's Degree) - University of Brasilia, 1984.

EGRY, E. Y. **Saude coletiva**: construindo um novo metodo em enfermagem. Sao Paulo: Icone, 1996.

ELIAS, M. A.; NAVARRO, V. L. The relationship between work, health and living conditions: negativity and positivity in the work of nursing professionals at a teaching hospital. **Revista Latino-americana de Enfermagem,** Ribeirao Preto, v. 14, n. 4, p. 517-525, 2006.

FACTS - European Agency for Safety and Health at Work. **How to tackle psychosocial risks and reduce stress at work**. 2002. Available at: <http://agency.osha.eu.int/publications/reports/index_en.htm>. Accessed on: May 12, 2014.

FARIAS, S. N. P.; MAURO, M. Y. C.; ZEITOUNE, R. C. G. Legal issues on the health of nursing workers. **Revista de Enfermagem da UERJ**, Rio de Janeiro, v. 8, n. 1, p. 28-32, 2000.

FERRAREZE, M. V. G.; FERREIRA, V.; CARVALHO, A. M. P. Perception of stress among intensive care nurses. **Acta Paulista de Enfermagem**, Sao Paulo, v. 19, n. 3, p. 310-315, feb. 2006.

FERRAZ, C.A. **Construindo uma pratica administrativa de enfermagem**, 1990. (mimeographed)

FIAMONCINI, R. L.; FIAMONCINI, R. E. Stress and muscle fatigue: factors affecting the quality of life of individuals. **Revista Digital**, v. 9, n. 66, 2003.

FLACH, L.; et al. Psychic suffering in contemporary work: analyzing a business magazine. **Psicologia & Sociedade**, Florianopolis, v. 21, n. 2, p.193-202, 2009.

FOUCAULT, M. **Microfisica do poder**. 11 ed. Rio de Janeiro: Graal, 1993.

FRANQA, F. M. de.; FERRARI, R. Chronic occupational stress and the sector in which hospital nursing professionals work. **Revista Eletrdnica Gestao & Saude** [internet], v. 03, n. 01, 531-545, 2012. Available at: <http://gestaoesaude.bce.unb.br/index.php/gestaoesaude/article/view/153/pdf_1>. Accessed on: Aug. 11, 2015.

GALLAR, M. **Promocion de la salud y apoyo psicologico al paciente**. Madrid: Paraninfo, 1998.

GELBCKE, F. L. **Health-disease process and work process: the view of nursing workers in a teaching hospital**. 1991.266f. Dissertation (Master's in Nursing) University of Rio de Janeiro, Rio de Janeiro, 1991.

GIOMO, D. B.; et al. Work accidents, occupational risks and absenteeism among hospital nursing workers. **Revista de enfermagem da UERJ**, Rio de Janeiro, v. 17, p. 24-29, 2009.

GIOVANINI, T. **Historia da enfermagem: versoes e interpretagoes**. Rio de Janeiro, Revinter, p. 205, 1995.

GIR, E.; et al. Accident with biological material and vaccination against hepatitis B among undergraduate students in the health area. **Revista Latino-America de Enfermagem**, Ribeirao Preto, v. 16, n. 3, p. 401-406, 2008.

GOMES, S. B. S. **Changes in the levels of self-image and self-esteem in physical education students through the application of a special postural gymnastics program.** 1997. 128f. Dissertation (Master's Degree) - School of Physical Education, Federal University of Rio Grande do Sul, Porto Alegre, 1997.

GOMES, R. A. Violence as a health problem for girls living on the streets. **Cadernos de Saude Publica**, Rio de Janeiro, v. 10, n. 1, p.156-167, 1994.

GUIDO, L. A. **Stress and coping among anesthesia recovery center nurses**. 2003. Thesis (Doctorate). School of Nursing - University of Sao Paulo, Sao Paulo, 2003.

HALL, L. A. et al. Self-esteem as a mediator of the effects of stressors and social resources on depressive symptoms in postpartum mothers. **Nursing Res**, United States, v. 45, p. 231-38, 1996.

HOGA, L. A. K. Causes of stress and mechanisms of well-being production in neonatal unit nursing professionals. **Acta Paulista de Enfermagem**, Sao Paulo, v.15, n. 2, p.18-25, 2002.

JUAREZ-GARCIA, A. Factores psicosociales laborales relacionados con la tensión arterial y sintomas cardiovasculares en personal de enfermeiro en Mexico. **Salud publica Mexico**, v.49, n.2, p. 109-117, 2007.

KAMIMURA, Q. P.; TAVARES, R. S. C. R. Accidents at Work Related to Occupational Psychological Disorders. **Revista de Gestao em Sistemas de Saude - RGSS**, Sao Paulo, v. 1, n. 2, p. 140-156, jul./dez. 2012.

KRANE, L.; et al. Attitudes towards sickness absence and sickness presenteeism in health and care sectors in Norway and Denmark: a qualitative study. **BMC Public Health**, London, v. 14, n. 880, p. 27, 2014.

LABRADOR, F. J. **Stress**. Madrid: Ediciones Temas de Hoy. S. A., 1992.

LANCMAN, S.; SZNELWAR, L. I. **Chistophe Dejours: da psicopatologia a psicodinamica do trabalho**. Editora Fiocruz, Brasilia, 2004.

LAURELL A. C.; NORIEGA, M. **Processo de produpao e saude:** trabalho e desgaste operario. Hucitec, Sao Paulo, 1989.

LAZARUS, R. S.; FOLKMAN, S. **Passion and reason.** New York: Oxford University Press, 1994.

LEE, G.; SHEHAN, C. L. Social relations and the selfesteem of older persons. **Reserch on Aging**, Durhan, v.11, n. 4, p. 427-442, 1989.

LEITAO, I. M. T. A.; FERNANDES, A. L.; RAMOS, I. C. Saude ocupacional: analisando os riscos relacionados a equipe de enfermagem numa unidade de terapia intensiva. **Ciencia Cuidado e Saude,** Maringa, v. 7, n. 4, p. 476-484, 2008.

LEOPARDI, M. T. et al. **The health work process**: organization and subjectivity. Florianopolis: Papa-livros, 1999. p. 39-41.

LIMA, F. A.; PINHEIRO, P. N. C.; VIEIRA, N. F. C. Accidents with sharps: understanding the feelings and emotions of nursing professionals. **Escola Anna Nery Revista de Enfermagem**, Rio de Janeiro, v. 11, n. 2, p. 205-211,2007.

LIPP, M. et al. Stress: basic concepts. **Research on stress in Brazil**. Campinas: Papirus, 1996.

MACHADO, M. R. M.; MACHADO, F. A. Accidents involving biological material among nursing workers at Palmas general hospital. **Revista Brasileira de Saude Ocupacional,** v. 36, n. 124, p. 274-281,2011.

MASLOW, A. H. **Motivation and personality**. Sagitario, 1 ed. Barcelona, 1954.

MARZIALE, M. H. P. **Ergonomic conditions of the working situation of nursing staff in a hospitalization unit**. 1995. 154 f. Thesis (Doctorate in Nursing). Ribeirao Preto Nursing School, University of Sao Paulo, Ribeirao Preto, 1995.

. Scientific production on occupational accidents with sharp materials among nursing workers. **Revista Latino-America de Enfermagem**, Ribeirao Preto, v. 10, n. 4, p. 81-85, 2002.

. Contributions of the occupational nurse in the promotion of workers' health. **Acta Paulista de Enfermagem**, Sao Paulo, v. 23, n. 2, Apr. 2010.

MAURO, M. Y. C. Saude mental do trabalhador e enfermeiro. **Revista de Enfermagem da UERJ**, Rio de Janeiro, v. 10, n. 1, p. 81-87, jan./abr. 1993.

MAURO, M. Y. C. et al. Nursing working conditions in the wards of a university hospital. **Escola Anna Nery Revista de Enfermagem**, Rio de Janeiro, v. 14, n. 1, p. 13-18, Apr./Jun. 2010.

MAURO, M. Y. C.; VEIGA, A. R. Health problems and occupational risks: perceptions of nursing workers in a maternal-child unit. **Revista de Enfermagem da UERJ**, Rio de Janeiro, v. 16, p. 64-69, 2008.

McGRATH, J. E. **Social and psychological factors in stress**. New York: Holt, Rinehart and Winston, 1970.

MECCA, A.; SMELSER, N. J.; VASCONCELLOS, J. **The social importance of selfesteem. Berkeley**. CA: University of California Press, 1989.

MELEK, T. H. R.; ROCHA, P. R. S. Enfermagem: tecendo fios historicos no contexto da sociedade global. **Revista Eletrdnica de Enfermagem do UNIERO**, Brasilia, v.1, n.1, p. 64-79, jan./abr. 2008.

MENDES, A. M. O. C. **Stress and immunity**: a contribution to the study of personal factors in stress-related immune alterations. Coimbra: Formasau, 2002.

MERLO, A. R. **Work Process and Health: An Introduction to the Theme.** Rio de Janeiro

Janeiro, ABRASCO (mimeo), 1991.

MICHEL, O. **Accidentes do trabalho e doengas ocupacionais**. Sao Paulo: LTR, 2000.

MININEL, V. A.; BABTISTA, P. C. P.; FELLI, V. E. A. Psychic burdens and stress processes in nursing workers in Brazilian university hospitals.
Revista Latino-americana de Enfermagem, Ribeirao Preto, v. 19, n. 2, mar./abr. 2011.

NATIONAL INSTITUTE FOR OCCUPATIONAL SAFETY AND HEALTH. **Guidelines for protecting the safety and health care workers** [online]. Atlanta; 1988. Available at: <http:// www.cdc.gov/niosh/hcwold1.html>. Accessed on: 07 Sep. 2013.

NAVARRO, V. L.; PADILHA, V. Dilemmas of work in contemporary capitalism. Psychol. Soc., Porto Alegre, v. 19, n. spe, 2007.

NEVES, M. J. A. O.; et al. Influência do trabalho nocturno na qualidade de vida do enfermeiro, **Revista de Enfermagem,** Rio de Janeiro, v. 18, n. 1, p. 42-47, jan./mar. 2010.

NISHIDE, V. M.; BENATTI, M. C. C. Occupational risks among nursing workers in an intensive care unit. **Revista da Escola de Enfermagem da USP**, Sao Paulo, v. 38, n. 4, p. 406-414, 2004.

NOBEN, C. Y.; et al. Quality appraisal of generic self-reported instruments measuring health-related productivity changes: a systematic review. **BMC Public Health**, London, v. 14, n. 115, p. 2-21,2014.

NUNES, M. B. G. **Occupational risks in the work of nurses working in the Basic Health Care Network in the Municipality of Volta Redonda-RJ**. 2009. Thesis (Doctorate in Nursing) - Ribeirao Preto School of Nursing, University of Sao Paulo, Ribeirao Preto, 2009.

INTERNATIONAL LABOR ORGANIZATION. **Factores psicosociales en el trabajo**. Geneva: International Labor Office; 1986.

OLIVEIRA, J. D. S. et al. Social representations of nurses about work stress in an emergency service. **Revista da Escola de Enfermagem USP**, Sao Paulo, v. 47, n. 4, p. 984-989, 2013.

WHO. World Health Organization. From old occupational medicine to new occupational health. **Revista Brasileira de Saude Ocupacional**, Sao Paulo, v. 114, n. 31, p. 112-118, 1999.

OGUISSO, T.; FREITAS G. F. Teaching and research on the history of nursing in undergraduate and graduate programs at the University of São Paulo School of Nursing. **Revista de Pesquisa: cuidado e fundamental,** Rio de Janeiro, v. 9, n. 1/2, p. 79-91, 2005.

PAIXAO, W. **Historia da enfermagem**. 5. ed. Rio de Janeiro: Julio C. Reis, 1979.

PIRES, J. C. S.; MACEDO, K. B. Organizational culture in public organizations in Brazil. Rev. Adm. Publica, Rio de Janeiro, v.40, n.1, p. 81-105, 2006.

PLACCO, V. M. N. S. Preface. In: TAVARES, J. (Org.) **Resilience and education**. Sao Paulo: Cortez, p. 7-12, 2001.

PROCHASKA, J. O. et al. **Journal of Occupational and Environmental Medicine**, v. 53, n. 7, p. 735-42, 2011.

QUIALA, M. F.; RODRIGUEZ, I. Z. Autoestima en el personal de enfermeria. **Revista Cubana de Enfermeria**, Habana, v. 15, n. 3, p. 184-189, 1999.

RANGEL, F. B. Psychosomatic symptoms and work organization: a study in an HEI. 2009, Sao Paulo. **Anais...** Sao Paulo, 2009.

RIBEIRO, E. J. G.; SHIMIZU, H. E. Work accidents involving nursing workers. **Revista Brasileira de Enfermagem** [Internet], v. 60, n. 5, Sept./Oct. 2007. Available at: <http://www.scielo.br/ pdf/reben/v60n5/v60n5a10.pdf>. Accessed on: 08 Aug 2015.

REINHOLD, H. H. **Analysis of scientific production at a Brazilian stress congress**. Available at: <http://www.estresse.com.br>. Accessed on: July 30, 2011.

ROBAZZI, M. L. C. C.; MARZIALE, M. H. P. Alguns problemas ocupacionais decorrentes do trabalho de enfermagem no Brasil. **Revista Brasileira de**

Enfermagem, Brasilia, v. 52, n. 3, p. 331-338, 1999.

ROBAZZI, M. L. C. C.; BARROS JUNIOR, J. C. Brazilian proposal for standardization for health workers. **Ciencia y Enfermeria** [on line], v. 11, n. 1, p. 1115, 2005. Available at: http://www.scielo.cl/pdf/cienf/v11n2/art03.pdf. Accessed: July 25, 2015.

ROCHA, G. V. M. **Analise da relagao entre praticas parentales e o autoconceito de pre-escolarares** (Dissertation). Postgraduate Program in Childhood and Adolescence Psychology, Federal University of Paraná, Curitiba, PR, 2002.

RONSEIN, G. E.; et al. Influence of stress on blood levels of lipids, ascorbic acid, zinc and other biochemical parameters. **Acta Bioquim. Clin. Latino Am.** La Plata, v. 38, n.1,2004.

ROSENBERG, M. **Society and the adolescent self-image**. New Jersey: Princeton University Press, 1965.

. **Society and the adolescent self-image**. Princeton, NJ: Princeton University Press, 1989 (Original published in 1956).

. **The Rosenberg self-Esteem Scale**. Available at: <http://www.bsos.umd.edu/socy/rosenberg.html>. Accessed on: May 17, 2014.

ROSSI, A. M.; MEURS, J. A.; PERREWE, P. L. (Organizers). Stress and quality of life at work: improving employee health and well-being. Sao Paulo: Atlas, 2013. 211 p.

RUIZ, M.T.; BARBOZA, D.B.; SOLER, Z. A. S. G. Accidents at work: a study on this occurrence in a general hospital. **Revista Arquivos de Ciencias da Saude**, v. 11, n. 4, p. 219-224, Oct./Dec. 2004.

SABBI, D. **Sinto, logo existo**. Porto Alegre: Alcance, 1999.

SADIR, M. A.; LIPP, M. E. N. Sources of stress at work. **Revista de Psicologia da Imed**, Passo Fundo, v. 1, n. 1, p. 114-126, 2009.

SAMULSKI, D. M. **Psicologia do Esporte.** Sao Paulo: Editora Manole, 2002. p. 380.

SANTANA, V. S. et al. Accidents at work: social security costs and working days lost. **Revista de Saude Publica**, Sao Paulo, v. 40, n. 6, p. 1004-1012, 2006.

SANTANA, L .L.; et al. Workload and stress experienced by health workers in a teaching hospital. **Revista Gaucha de Enfermagem**, Porto Alegre, v. 34, n. 1, p. 64-70, 2013.

SANTOS, J. M.; OLIVEIRA, E. B.; MOREIRA, A. C. Estresse, fator de risco para a saude do enfermeiro em Centro de Terapia Intensiva. **Revista de Enfermagem da UERJ**,Rio de Janeiro, v. 14, n. 4, p. 580-585, Oct./Dec. 2006.

SCHIEMAN, S.; CAMPBELL, J. E. Age variations in personal agency and selfesteem: the context of physical disability. **Journal of Aging and Health**, London, v. 13, n. 2, p. 155-185, 2001.

SCHMIDT, D. R. C. **Quality of life at work and its association with occupational stress, physical and mental health and sense of coherence among nursing professionals in the operating room**. 2009. Thesis (PhD) - Ribeirao Preto School of Nursing, University of Sao Paulo, Ribeirao Preto, 2009.

SECCO, I. A. O. et al. Psychic workloads and burnout of nursing workers at a teaching hospital in Paraná, Brazil. **Revista Eletrdnica Saude Mental Alcool e Drogas**, Ribeirao Preto, v. 6, n.1, p. 1-17, 2010.

SERRA, A. V. **O stress na vida de todos os dias**. 2. ed. Coimbra, 2002.
SELYE, H. A syndrome produced by diverse nocuous agents. **Nature**, v.138, p. 32, 1936.

. **The stress of life**. New York: McGraw-Hill, 1956.

SHIMIZU, H. E; CIAMPONE, M. H. T. Suffering and pleasure at work experienced by nurses working in Intensive Care Units in a teaching hospital. **Rev Esc. Enferm. USP**. Sao Paulo, v. 33, n.1, p. 95-106, 1999.

SILVA, C. D. L.; PINTO, W. M. Occupational risks in the hospital environment: factors that favor their occurrence in the nursing team. **Saude Coletiva em Debate**, Sao Paulo, v. 2, n. 1, p. 62-69, dec. 2012.

SILVA, G. **Enfermagem profissional analise critica**. 2 ed. Sao Paulo, SP: Cortez; 1989.

SILVA, L. A. da. **Environmental exposure to carbon monoxide and accidents at work among motorcycle taxi drivers: a contribution from occupational nursing**. 2012. 203f. Thesis (Doctorate in Nursing). Ribeirao Preto School of Nursing, University of Sao Paulo, Ribeirao Preto, 2012.

SILVA NETO, J. P.; ALEXANDRE, S. M. B.; SOUSA, M. N. A. de. Accidents at work and underreporting: a study of nurses working in tertiary care. **C&D- Revista Eletrdnica da Fainor,** Vitoria da Conquista, v.7, n.2, p.219-231, jul./dez. 2014.

SILVA, N. F. A.; LIMA, M. J. O. Qualidade de vida no trabalho: o estudo qualitativo na empresa natura. *In:* V Semana cientifica e cultural do Servipo Social das Faculdades Unificadas da Fundapao Educacional de Barretos, 2007, Barretos. **Proceedings...** Barretos: FUFEB, 2007.

SILVA, V. E. F. **The wear and tear of the nursing worker: the relationship between nursing work and workers' health**. 1996, 189 f. Thesis (Doctorate in Nursing) - School of Nursing, University of Sao Paulo, Sao Paulo, 1996.

SIMAO, S. A. F.; et al. Work accidents with sharps involving nursing professionals in a hospital emergency unit. **Revista de enfermagem da UERJ**, Rio de Janeiro, v. 18, n. 3, p. 400-404, jul./set. 2010.

SOARES, R. S.; et al. Accidents with sharps in the nursing team. **Revista de Pesquisa e Cuidado Fundamental Online**, (Suppl): p. 1-4, 2012.

SOUTO, D. F. Gases and Vapors in the Workplace. **Brazilian Society of Safety Engineering**, 2005. Available at: <http://www.sobes.org.br/Figuras/gases.pdf.>. Accessed on: 13 Aug 2015.

SOUZA E SILVA, R. **Transformations in the world of work, unemployment and their impact on the organization of Brazilian workers**. 2008. Course Conclusion Paper - School of Social Work - Center for Philosophy and Human Sciences, University of Rio de Janeiro, Rio de Janeiro, 2008.

SOUSA, I. F.; MENDONQA, H. Burnout in University Professors: Impact of Perceptions of Justice and Affective Commitment. **Pic. Teor. Pesq.** ,Brasilia, v. 25, n.4, p. 499-508, 2009.

STACCIARINI, J. M. R.; TROCCOLI, B. T. Instrument for measuring occupational stress: the nurses' stress inventory (IEE). **Rev. latino-am. enfermagem**, Ribeirao Preto, v. 8, n. 6, p. 40-49, 2000.

STUMM, E. M. F. **The stress of nursing teams working in Surgical Center Units in Hospitals in the City of Ijui**. 2000.
Dissertation (Master's Degree) - Federal University of Rio Grande do Sul, Postgraduate Program in Administration, Porto Alegre, 2000.

TAMAYO, A.; CUNHA, P. Self-concept, sex and frequency of premarital sexual activity. **Ciencia e Cultura,** Campinas, v. 35, n. 7, 1983.

TERRA, F.S. **Evaluation of anxiety, depression and self-esteem in nursing professors from public and private universities**. 2010, 258f. Thesis (Doctorate in Nursing), Ribeirao Preto Nursing School, University of Sao Paulo, Ribeirao Preto, SP, 2010.

TIRONI, M. O. S.; et al. Work and Burnout Syndrome in intensive care physicians in Salvador. **Rev. Assoc. Med. Bras.**, v. 55, n. 6, p. 656-62, 2009.

THE WHOQOL GROUP. The World Health Organization quality of life assessment (WHOQOL): position paper from the World Health Organization. **Social Science and Medicine,** v. 10, p. 1403-1409, 1995.

TONINI, N. S.; FLEMING, S. F. Nursing history: evolution and research. **Revista Arquivos de Ciencias da Saude**, v. 6, n. 3, Sept./Dec. 2002.

TREVIZAN, M. A. **Enfermagem hospitalar: administrapao & burocracia**. Brasilia: Ed. UnB, 1988.

TURKIEWICZ, M. **History of nursing**. ETECLA, 1995.

VALIM, M. D.; MARZIALE, M. H. P. Evaluation of occupational exposure to biological material in health services. **Texto e contexto Enfermagem**, Florianopolis, v. 20 - Special p.138-146, 2011.

VARGAS, T. V. P.; DANTAS, R. A. S.; GOIS, C. F. L. The self-esteem of individuals who have undergone coronary artery bypass graft surgery. **Revista Escola Enfermagem da USP**, Sao Paulo, v. 39, n. 1, p. 20-27, 2005.

VELASCO, A. R. et al. Occurrence of occupational accidents in health with exposure to biological material. **Revista de Enfermagem Profissional**, Rio de Janeiro, v. 1, n. 1, p. 37-49, jan./abr. 2014.

VIEIRA, S. I.; SCHULLER SOBRINHO, O. **Estresse e sua Prevenpao**. Coord: VIEIRA, S. I. In: **Medicina Basica do Trabalho**. v. 4, Curitiba: Genesis, 1995. p. 199 - 217.

VIEIRA, T. G. et al. Illness and use of psychoactive drugs among nursing workers in intensive care units. **Revista de Enfermagem da UFSM**, Santa Maria, v. 3, n. 2, p. 205-214, mai./ago. 2013.

VITORIA REGIS, L. F. L.; PORTO I. S. The nursing team and Maslow: (in) Satisfactions at work. **Revista Brasileira de Enfermagem**, Brasilia, v. 59, n. 4, p. 565-568, 2006.

WADA, K.; et al. The economic impact of loss of performance due to absenteeism and presenteeism caused by depressive symptoms and comorbid health conditions among Japanese workers. **Industrial Health**, Tokyo, v. 51, n. 5, p. 482-489, 2013.

ZEITLIN, L. R. Organizational Downsizing and stress-related illness. **International Journal of Stress Management**, v. 2, n. 4, p. 207-220, 1995.

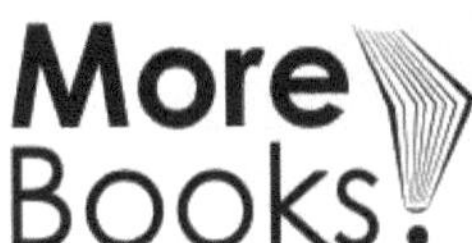

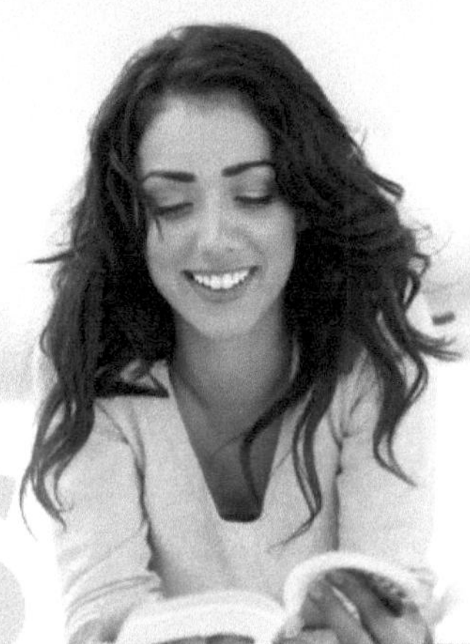

yes
I want morebooks!

Buy your books fast and straightforward online - at one of world's fastest growing online book stores! Environmentally sound due to Print-on-Demand technologies.

Buy your books online at
www.morebooks.shop

Kaufen Sie Ihre Bücher schnell und unkompliziert online – auf einer der am schnellsten wachsenden Buchhandelsplattformen weltweit! Dank Print-On-Demand umwelt- und ressourcenschonend produzi ert.

Bücher schneller online kaufen
www.morebooks.shop

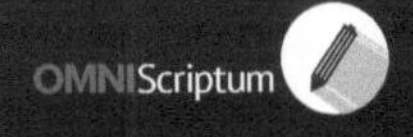

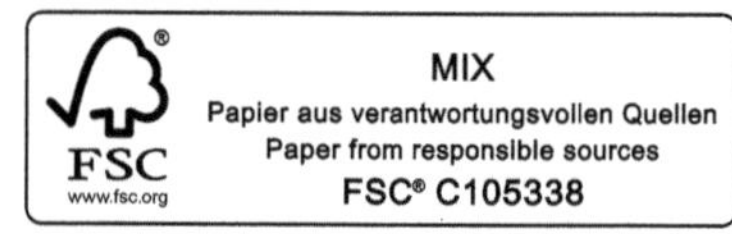

Printed by Books on Demand GmbH, Norderstedt / Germany